New Perspectives in Behavioral & Health Sciences

New Perspectives in Behavioral & Health Sciences is a series of high-quality, compact volumes focused on presenting interdisciplinary perspectives on key, developing, or new topics in Behavioral and Health Sciences. This SpringerBrief series will be of interest to a broad range of researchers and practitioners working in related fields of Behavioral and Health Sciences such as Psychology, Mental Health, Criminology, Public Health, and Social Work.

Gabriel Bennett

Autistic People in Dental and Medical Clinics

Challenges and Solutions

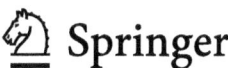 Springer

Gabriel Bennett
Independent Researcher
Adelaide, SA, Australia

ISSN 2731-9296   ISSN 2731-930X (electronic)
New Perspectives in Behavioral & Health Sciences
ISBN 978-981-99-2358-8   ISBN 978-981-99-2359-5 (eBook)
https://doi.org/10.1007/978-981-99-2359-5

This Springer imprint is published by the registered company Springer Nature Singapore Pte Ltd.
The registered company address is: 152 Beach Road, #21-01/04 Gateway East, Singapore 189721,
Singapore

I dedicate this book to future generations of medical and dental professionals who will assist autistics and their families.

About This Book

Undergoing medical and dental examinations and treatment can be a daunting experience for autistics. Combining the perspectives of autistic patients, their parents, and medical professionals, *Autistic People in Dental and Medical Clinics: Challenges and Solutions* is a groundbreaking book that sheds light on the experiences and needs of autistic patients in medical and dental clinics. It highlights the barriers that exist in these settings, such as sensory sensitivities, communication difficulties, and a lack of understanding about the autism spectrum by healthcare providers. It also outlines strategies for improving the experiences of autistic patients in medical and dental clinics. Whether you are autistic, a medical professional, or a caregiver, this book is a must-read for anyone looking to improve the healthcare experiences of autistic participants.

Choice of Terminology

There is an ongoing debate in the field of autism spectrum research, as well as in the broader field of disability studies, as to what is the most appropriate use of terminology to address members of the autistic community (Tepest, 2021; Vivanti, 2020). Some prefer using person-first language (i.e., people on the autism spectrum) while others prefer using identity-first language (i.e., autistic person). Throughout this book, I use identity-first language since contemporary research has shown that most autistics prefer this language convention (Bury et al., 2023; Kenny et al., 2016). Furthermore, it is my belief, as an autistic researcher, that since the autism spectrum is an inseparable part of a person's identity that the word *'autistic'* should be used instead of *'person with autism'* or *'person on the autism spectrum'*.

References

Bury, S. M., Jellett, R., Spoor, J. R., & Hedley, D. (2023). "It defines who I am" or "it's something I have": What language do [autistic] Australian adults [on the autism spectrum] prefer? *Journal of Autism and Developmental Disorders. 53*(2), 677–687. https://doi.org/10.1007/s10803-020-04425-3

Kenny, L., Hattersley, C., Molins, B., Buckley, C., Povey, C., & Pellicano, E. (2016). Which terms should be used to describe autism? Perspectives from the UK autism community. *Autism: The International Journal of Research and Practice, 20*(4), 442–462. https://doi.org/10.1177/1362361315588200

Tepest, R. (2021). The meaning of diagnosis for different designations in talking about autism. *Journal of Autism and Developmental Disorders, 51*(2), 760–761. https://doi.org/10.1007/s10803-020-04584-3

Vivanti, G. (2020). Ask the editor: What is the most appropriate way to talk about individuals with a diagnosis of autism? *Journal of Autism and Developmental Disorders, 50*(2), 691–693. https://doi.org/10.1007/s10803-019-04280-x

Contents

About the Author

Dr. Gabriel Bennett Ph.D., the pen name for Dr. Matthew Bennett Ph.D., is an autistic researcher who examines various aspects of the autism spectrum. He believes that one of the best ways to improve the lives of autistics is through the creation and dissemination of knowledge that has translational benefits for the autistic community. He has published several books about the autism spectrum, including:

1. Bennett, M., Webster, A. A., Goodall, E., & Rowland, S. (2019). *Life on the autism spectrum: Translating myths and misconceptions into positive futures.* Springer. https://doi.org/10.1007/978-981-13-3359-0
2. Bennett, M., Goodall, E., & Nugent, J. (2020). *Choosing Effective Support for People on the Autism Spectrum: A Guide Based on Academic Perspectives and Lived Experience.* Routledge. https://doi.org/10.4324/9780367821975
3. Bennett, M., & Goodall, E. (2021). *Sexual Behaviours and Relationships of Autistics: A Scoping Review.* Springer International Publishing AG. https://doi.org/10.1007/978-3-030-65599-0
4. Bennett, M., & Goodall, E. (2021). *Employment of Persons with Autism: A Scoping Review.* Springer International Publishing AG. https://doi.org/10.1007/978-3-030-82174-6
5. Bennett, M., & Goodall, E. (2022). *Addressing Underserved Populations in Autism Spectrum Research: An Intersectional Approach.* Emerald Publishing Group. https://doi.org/10.1108/9781803824635
6. Bennett, M., & Goodall, E. (2022). *Autism and COVID-19: Strategies for Supporters to Help Autistics and Their Families.* Emerald Publishing Group. https://doi.org/10.1108/9781804550335

List of Abbreviations

MEPS   Medical Expenditure Panel Survey
NHIS   National Health Interview Survey
PRISMA   Preferred Reporting Items for Systematic Reviews and Meta-Analyses

List of Figures

List of Tables

Chapter 1
Introduction

1.1 Autistics in Healthcare

There has been a consistent increase each year in the number of studies about autism since Dr Leo Kanner's paper about the condition, titled '*Autistic disturbances of affective contact*' (Kanner, 1943). This point can be illustrated by a search of PubMed with the word '*autism*' in the article's title (see Fig. 1.1). This yearly increase should be applauded since it has given us an abundance of knowledge about autism and what it can be like to be autistic.

Along with other insights, the increased volume of literature about autism has revealed that autistics typically have more physical, dental, and mental health problems compared to non-autistics (Forde et al., 2022) (see Appendix 1.1). This volume of literature has also shown that autistics often have a greater need for medical and dental services. Despite requiring more support from the healthcare system, autistics usually have difficulties accessing and navigating this system. Exacerbating these difficulties is the lack of knowledge that medical and dental professionals have about treating autistic patients (Adams & Young, 2020; Calleja et al., 2020; Hossain et al., 2020; Lai et al., 2019). To help rectify this situation, it is vital that the healthcare system responds to the individualised needs of autistic patients. To achieve this objective, healthcare professionals should have a comprehensive understanding about the experiences of autistics in medical and dental settings from the perspective of autistics themselves, their families, and healthcare professionals who treat autistic patients. It is also crucial that healthcare professionals and policymakers comprehend some of the typical barriers that autistic patients encounter in the healthcare system and provide some evidence-based solutions to these barriers.

G. Bennett, *Autistic People in Dental and Medical Clinics*, New Perspectives in Behavioral & Health Sciences, https://doi.org/10.1007/978-981-99-2359-5_1

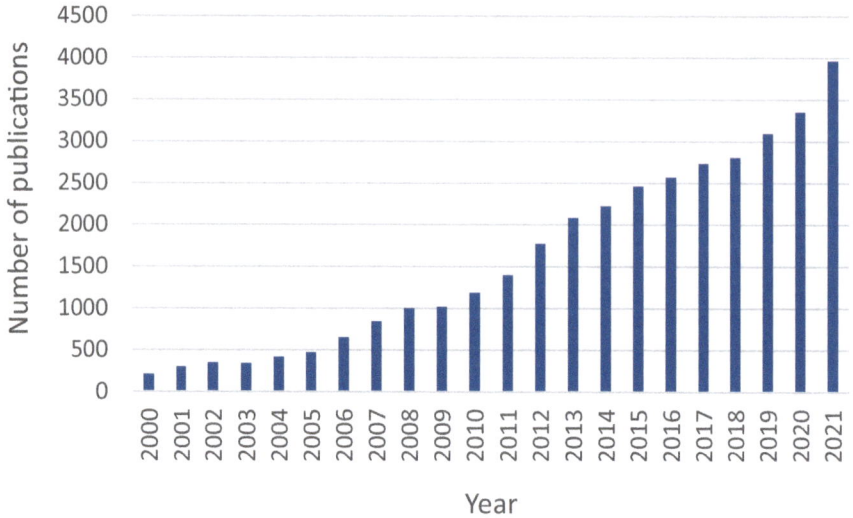

Fig. 1.1 Number of articles with the word '*autism*' in the article's title hosted on PubMed from 2000 to 2021*. *Search was conducted on 17 December 2022 using the search term '*autism*' in the article's title

There are studies about the experiences and barriers to accessing dental and medical systems from the perspective of autistics (Adams & Young, 2020). Regrettably, there is no contemporary synthesis of this literature. This study addresses this gap by answering the following research questions:

1. What experiences have autistics had in medical clinics?
2. What experiences have autistics had in dental clinics?
3. What experiences have dentists had with treating autistics?
4. What experiences have doctors had with treating autistics?
5. What experiences have parents had with their autistic child receiving dental care?
6. What experiences have parents had with their autistic child receiving medical care?
7. What barriers prevent autistics from receiving medical care?
8. What barriers prevent autistics from receiving dental care?
9. What strategies can be used to help autistics attend dental and medical clinics?

1.2   Search Procedures for Locating Suitable Literature

On 12 November 2022, four distinct searches of PubMed were conducted to identify studies about the experiences of autistics in medical and dental clinics. To be included in this book, the article had to have been published in English and had to have a sample of autistics and/or parents/caregivers of autistics and/or doctors and/or dentists. This

Table 1.1 Results from the PubMed search

Search permutation	Number of results
(autis*[Title]) AND (oral[Title])	87
(autis*[Title]) AND (dental[Title])	74
(autis*[Title]) AND (medical[Title])	85
(autis*[Title]) AND (healthcare[Title])	74
Total	320

general eligibility criteria ensured that the largest possible number of studies about the experiences of autistics in medical or dental settings retrieved from the four PubMed searches could be included in this study. All searches involved restricting the search terms to the article's title. All search combinations involved using the search term '*autis**'. The use of the asterisk (*) enabled different terms related to autism to also be searched, including '*autism*', '*autism spectrum*', '*autistic*', and '*autism spectrum disorder*'. Finally, articles that were published from 12 November 2018 to 12 November 2022 were only included. This date range ensured that only contemporary studies with the most recent insights were retrieved for examination. In total, 320 articles were retrieved and after 14 duplicate records were removed 306 original articles were examined (see Table 1.1).

A *Preferred Reporting Items for Systematic Reviews and Meta-Analyses* (PRISMA) analysis approach was used to examine the citations retrieved from the four PubMed searches. PRISMA is an established method for collecting, examining, and identifying suitable studies from a large sample of collected literature. PRISMA has been used to examine the literature about various aspects of the autism spectrum, including film and television representations of autistics (Dean & Nordahl-Hansen, 2022) and problematic Internet usage among autistic children, adolescents, and adults (Normand et al., 2022). The PRISMA analysis approach has five steps, which were:

1. *STEP 1*: The first step was searching PubMed for studies about the medical and dental experiences of autistic as well as such experiences from the perspectives of their families and healthcare professionals. This search process involved conducting four separate searches for studies hosted on PubMed, which were:

   (a)   (autis*[Title]) AND (oral[Title])
   (b)   (autis*[Title]) AND (dental[Title])
   (c)   (autis*[Title]) AND (medical[Title])
   (d)   (autis*[Title]) AND (healthcare[Title])

2. *STEP 2*: The second step involved removing any duplicate records that were retrieved from the four searches of PubMed. It was discovered that 14 citations were duplicates which, once removed, meant that there were 306 original citations.

3. *STEP 3*: The third step involved examining each study's title and abstract to determine if it met the study's eligibility criteria and answered any of the nine

research questions. Of the 306 original citations that were examined, 33 were deemed to be of interest.

4. *STEP 4*: The fourth step involved reading the entire text of the 33 studies that were provisionally judged to be of relevance to the study. However, three studies could not be retrieved. This full-text examination of the remaining 30 studies resulted in all 30 being deemed to answer one or more of the study's nine research questions. Characteristics of these studies (e.g., the study's limitations, the sample size in the study) were identified and documented on an '*evaluation form*' (see Appendix 1.2). This form enabled a simple collation of different information about the study and a quick and easy comparison between included studies.

5. *STEP 5*: The fifth and final step involved examining and presenting results from the 30 studies that were retained from the fourth step in the PRISMA analysis process (see Fig. 1.2).

1.3   Limitations of This Study

1.3.1   *No Examination of the Mental Health System*

Autistics have mental health issues and their difficulties with accessing the mental health system have been acknowledged by autistics and professionals in the mental health system (Camm-Crosbie et al., 2019; Coleman-Fountain et al., 2020; Crane et al., 2019; Maddox et al., 2020). For brevity, this topic and strategies to help autistic enter the mental health system are not explored in this study.

1.3.2   *Date Limitations on the Articles Included*

Any studies published before 12 November 2018 were excluded to ensure that the most contemporary literature about autistics receiving medical and dental treatment was examined. Consequently, studies published before 12 November 2018, such as Nicolaidis and colleagues (2015) and Raymaker and colleagues (2017), that could have provided additional insights were not examined.

1.3.3   *Only Accessing Studies from PubMed*

All articles examined for this study were obtained from four separate searches of PubMed that occurred on 12 November 2022.

However, despite its benefits, PubMed did not index all relevant studies. For example, articles published by the journal *Review Journal of Autism and Developmental Disorders*, such as Corden et al.'s (2022) paper '*A Systematic Review of*

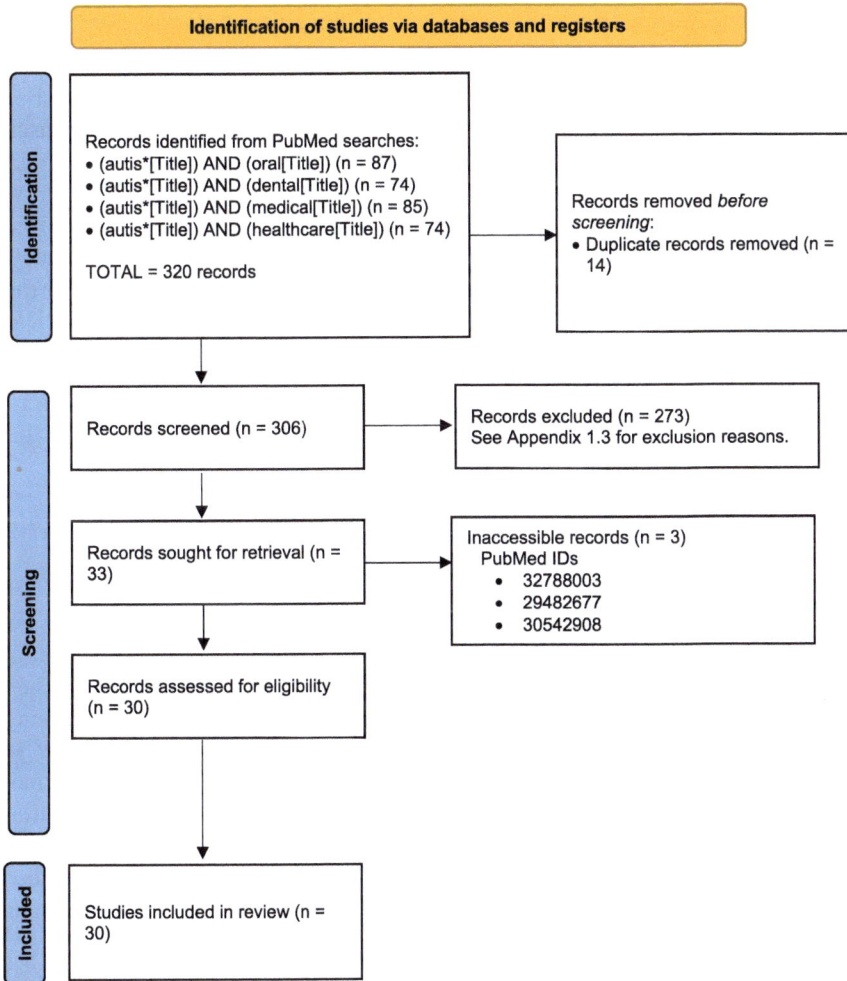

Fig. 1.2 Preferred reporting items for systematic reviews and meta-analyses (PRISMA) flow diagram. *Source* Page, M. J., McKenzie, J. E., Bossuyt, P. M., Boutron, I., Hoffmann, T. C., Mulrow, C. D., Shamseer, L., Tetzlaff, J. M., Akl, E. A., Brennan, S. E., Chou, R., Glanville, J., Grimshaw, J. M., Hróbjartsson, A., Lalu, M. M., Li, T., Loder, E. W., Mayo-Wilson, E., McDonald, S., McGuinness, L. A., … Moher, D. (2021). The PRISMA 2020 statement: An updated guideline for reporting systematic reviews. *BMJ (Clinical research ed.), 372*, n71. https://doi.org/10.1136/bmj.n71

Healthcare Professionals' Knowledge, Self-Efficacy and Attitudes Towards Working with Autistic People', were not indexed on PubMed. Thus, some articles were not collected and examined.

1.3.4 Restricting the Search Terms to Only the Article's Title

Four separate searches of PubMed were conducted to locate relevant studies about the needs and experiences of autistics in both medical and dental clinics. To ensure that the most relevant studies were discovered, the article's title had to contain one of the following search terms 'autism', 'autism spectrum', 'autistic', and 'autism spectrum disorder'. Despite its efficiency, it is possible that some articles were not retrieved from PubMed using this approach because the search term was embedded within the article's full text instead of its title. However, the prospect of this occurring was deemed to be negligible. Nevertheless, it cannot be ruled out that some articles may not have been identified.

1.4 Benefits of This Study

1.4.1 Publication of the Study's Dataset

The inability to validate existing results using the same dataset and methodology has undermined the certainty about the truthfulness of published results. This inability to validate results has been termed the 'reproducibility crisis' (Baker, 2016). There are many different factors that have contributed to this crisis, including p-hacking, confirmation bias, and publication bias. However, not publishing the study's dataset has contributed to this crisis. In the interests of reducing the possibility of this study succumbing to the reproducibility crisis, Appendix 1.3 lists all records retrieved from the four PubMed searches, along with justifications for why each study was either included or excluded from the analysis. By including this information, researchers can repeat the same analysis process to either confirm or challenge the conclusions reported.

1.4.2 Using PubMed

PubMed was the only database that was used to search for relevant research because, at the time of this book, it indexed more than 30 million records. PubMed was also used because it contained studies that were published by several reputable academic publishers, such as SAGE, Springer, and Taylor and Francis. Similarly, it contained studies published in reputable academic journals about the autism spectrum, such as the *Journal of Autism and Developmental Disorders* and *Autism: The International Journal of Research and Practice*. Due to its coverage, it was decided that searching PubMed was more efficient than conducting individual searches of reputable academic publishers.

1.5   Audience for This Book

This book has been written for many different audiences, including:

1. *Healthcare professionals*: Healthcare professionals, such as doctors, dentists, and nurses, will find this book useful for improving their ability to support autistic patients in their practices (Austriaco et al., 2019; Clarke & Fung, 2022; Low & Zailan, 2016; Mac Giolla Phadraig et al., 2022). For example, a dentist may learn about the use of visual aids to explain procedures and the importance of clear, concise communication with autistic patients.
2. *Family members and caregivers of autistics*: Family members and caregivers of autistics will find this book helpful for understanding how to better support their loved ones in medical and dental settings. For example, a parent of an autistic child may learn about strategies for reducing their child's anxiety during dental visits, such as the use of headphones to cancel out noise and a weighted blanket for comfort.
3. *Therapists*: Therapists may find this book useful for understanding how to support autistic clients in medical and dental settings. For example, a therapist may learn about ways to support autistic clients during medical procedures and the importance of clear, concise information about procedures.
4. *Autistic individuals and their advocates*: Some autistics have difficulties in medical and dental clinics (Calleja et al., 2020; Doherty et al., 2022; Junnarker et al., 2022; Mason et al., 2019; Mirsky et al., 2021; Weir et al., 2022). Autistics and their advocates may be interested in this book because they would learn about some ways to improve their experiences in medical and dental clinics. For example, autistics may learn about the importance of advocating for their needs in these settings and the use of accommodations, such as noise-cancelling headphones, to reduce sensory overload.
5. *Policymakers*: Policymakers and healthcare administrators may find this book useful for understanding the challenges that autistics encounter in medical and dental settings and developing policies to improve their experiences. For example, a healthcare administrator may learn about the need for clear, concise information about procedures and the use of accommodations to support autistic patients in medical and dental settings.

These are just a few examples of the different audiences who may be interested in reading this book. Ultimately, this book may be of interest to anyone who wants to learn about ways to better support and accommodate the needs of autistics in medical and dental clinics.

1.6   Benefits of This Book

This book will provide many benefits for the reader, including:

- *Increased understanding of autism*: The reader will learn about the common features associated with autism and how these features can impact autistics in different ways in medical and dental environments. For example, they may learn about the difficulties some autistics may experience with sensory overload in medical or dental environments and how to make accommodations to support them.
- *Improved communication skills*: This book will help readers learn about the communication difficulties that some autistics may encounter and strategies to support effective communication in a medical or dental setting. For example, they may learn about the importance of clear, concise language and avoiding overwhelming stimuli for autistic patients.
- *Improved empathy*: The reader will gain a deeper understanding of the experiences of autistics in medical and dental settings and how to support them. For example, they may learn about the anxiety that many autistic patients feel in these environments and how to make accommodations to reduce their stress.
- *Improved patient outcomes*: By learning about the specific needs and challenges of autistic patients, the reader will be better equipped to create a supportive and accommodating environment that can improve patient outcomes. For example, they may learn about the importance of providing clear, detailed information about procedures and the use of visual aids to support autistic patients.
- *Increased knowledge of accommodating technologies*: The reader will learn about technologies and accommodations that can support autistic patients in medical and dental settings, such as noise-cancelling headphones, weighted blankets, and iPad apps for distraction during procedures. By incorporating these accommodations into their practice, the reader would be better equipped to support the needs of autistic patients and improve their experiences in medical and dental environments.

1.7   Summary of Upcoming Chapters

1.7.1   Chapter 2—Autistics in Medical Settings

Chapter 2 contains a synthesis of literature about autistics in medical clinics. Embedded within this synthesis are the views of autistics, their parents, and medical practitioners about this topic. Additionally, gaps in our understanding about the literature examined are also explored. A series of suggestions that can help doctors treat autistic patients concludes this chapter.

1.7.2 Chapter 3—Autistics in Dental Clinics

Chapter 3 gives the reader an overview of the literature about autistics in dental settings. This overview includes the views of autistics, their family members, and professionals about providing dental care to autistics. Additionally, this chapter contains explanations about the limitations in our knowledge about autistics in dental settings. This chapter concludes with a series of suggestions that can help dentists treat autistic patients.

1.7.3 Chapter 4—Final Comments

Chapter 4 summarises the main points in this book and reiterates the gaps in our understanding about autistics in medical and dental clinics. Highlighting such gaps will help explain what research in the future could be conducted.

References

Adams, D., & Young, K. (2020). A systematic review of the perceived barriers and facilitators to accessing psychological treatment for mental health problems in individuals on the autism spectrum. *Review Journal of Autism and Developmental Disorders, 8*(4), 436–453. https://doi.org/10.1007/s40489-020-00226-7

Austriaco, K., Aban, I., Willig, J., & Kong, M. (2019). Contemporary trainee knowledge of autism: How prepared are our future providers? *Frontiers in Pediatrics, 7*, 165. https://doi.org/10.3389/fped.2019.00165

Baker, M. (2016). Reproducibility crisis. *Nature, 533*(26), 353–566. https://doi.org/10.1038/533452a

Calleja, S., Islam, F. M. A., Kingsley, J., & McDonald, R. (2020). Healthcare access for autistic adults: A systematic review. *Medicine, 99*(29), e20899. https://doi.org/10.1097/MD.0000000000020899

Camm-Crosbie, L., Bradley, L., Shaw, R., Baron-Cohen, S., & Cassidy, S. (2019). 'People like me don't get support': Autistic adults' experiences of support and treatment for mental health difficulties, self-injury and suicidality. *Autism: The International Journal of Research and Practice, 23*(6), 1431–1441. https://doi.org/10.1177/1362361318816053

Clarke, L., & Fung, L. K. (2022). The impact of autism-related training programs on physician knowledge, self-efficacy, and practice behavior: A systematic review. *Autism: The International Journal of Research and Practice, 26*(7), 1626–1640. https://doi.org/10.1177/13623613221102016

Coleman-Fountain, E., Buckley, C., & Beresford, B. (2020). Improving mental health in autistic young adults: A qualitative study exploring help-seeking barriers in UK primary care. *The British Journal of General Practice, 70*(694), e356–e363. https://doi.org/10.3399/bjgp20X709421

Corden, K., Brewer, R., & Cage, E. (2022). A systematic review of healthcare professionals' knowledge, self-efficacy and attitudes towards working with autistic people. *Review Journal of Autism and Developmental Disorders, 9*(3), 386–399. https://doi.org/10.1007/s40489-021-00263-w

Crane, L., Adams, F., Harper, G., Welch, J., & Pellicano, E. (2019). 'Something needs to change': Mental health experiences of young autistic adults in England. *Autism: The International Journal of Research and Practice, 23*(2), 477–493. https://doi.org/10.1177/1362361318757048

Dean, M., & Nordahl-Hansen, A. (2022). A review of research studying film and television representations of ASD. *Review Journal of Autism and Developmental Disorders, 9*(4), 470–479. https://doi.org/10.1007/s40489-021-00273-8

Doherty, M., Neilson, S., O'Sullivan, J., Carravallah, L., Johnson, M., Cullen, W., & Shaw, S. C. K. (2022). Barriers to healthcare and self-reported adverse outcomes for autistic adults: A cross-sectional study. *BMJ Open, 12*(2), e056904. https://doi.org/10.1136/bmjopen-2021-056904

Forde, J., Bonilla, P. M., Mannion, A., Coyne, R., Haverty, R., & Leader, G. (2022). Health status of adults with autism spectrum disorder. *Review Journal of Autism and Developmental Disorders, 9*(3), 427–437. https://doi.org/10.1007/s40489-021-00267-6

Hossain, M. M., Khan, N., Sultana, A., Ma, P., McKyer, E., Ahmed, H. U., & Purohit, N. (2020). Prevalence of comorbid psychiatric disorders among people with autism spectrum disorder: An umbrella review of systematic reviews and meta-analyses. *Psychiatry Research, 287*, 112922. https://doi.org/10.1016/j.psychres.2020.112922

Junnarkar, V. S., Tong, H. J., Hanna, K. M. B., Aishworiya, R., & Duggal, M. (2022). Occupational and speech therapists' perceptions of their role in dental care for children with autism spectrum disorder: A qualitative exploration. *International Journal of Paediatric Dentistry, 32*(6), 865–876. https://doi.org/10.1111/ipd.13009

Kanner, L. (1943). Autistic disturbances of affective contact. *Nervous Child, 2*(3), 217–250.

Lai, M. C., Kassee, C., Besney, R., Bonato, S., Hull, L., Mandy, W., Szatmari, P., & Ameis, S. H. (2019). Prevalence of co-occurring mental health diagnoses in the autism population: A systematic review and meta-analysis. *The Lancet Psychiatry, 6*(10), 819–829. https://doi.org/10.1016/S2215-0366(19)30289-5

Low, H. M., & Zailan, F. (2016). Medical students' perceptions, awareness, societal attitudes and knowledge of autism spectrum disorder: An exploratory study in Malaysia. *International Journal of Developmental Disabilities, 64*(2), 86–95. https://doi.org/10.1080/20473869.2016.1264663

Mac Giolla Phadraig, C., Kahatab, A., & Daly, B. (2022). Promoting openness to autism amongst dental care professional students. *European Journal of Dental Education: Official Journal of the Association for Dental Education in Europe, 27*(2), 396–401. https://doi.org/10.1111/eje.12821

Maddox, B. B., Crabbe, S., Beidas, R. S., Brookman-Frazee, L., Cannuscio, C. C., Miller, J. S., Nicolaidis, C., & Mandell, D. S. (2020). "I wouldn't know where to start": Perspectives from clinicians, agency leaders, and autistic adults on improving community mental health services for autistic adults. *Autism: The International Journal of Research and Practice, 24*(4), 919–930. https://doi.org/10.1177/1362361319882227

Mason, D., Ingham, B., Urbanowicz, A., Michael, C., Birtles, H., Woodbury-Smith, M., Brown, T., James, I., Scarlett, C., Nicolaidis, C., & Parr, J. R. (2019). A systematic review of what barriers and facilitators prevent and enable physical healthcare services access for autistic adults. *Journal of Autism and Developmental Disorders, 49*(8), 3387–3400. https://doi.org/10.1007/s10803-019-04049-2

Mirsky, L. B., Rogo, E. J., & Gurenlian, J. R. (2021). Oral care experiences of young adults with autism spectrum disorder. *Journal of Dental Hygiene, 95*(4), 41–50.

Nicolaidis, C., Raymaker, D. M., Ashkenazy, E., McDonald, K. E., Dern, S., Baggs, A. E., Kapp, S. K., Weiner, M., & Boisclair, W. C. (2015). "Respect the way I need to communicate with you": Healthcare experiences of adults on the autism spectrum. *Autism: The International Journal of Research and Practice, 19*(7), 824–831. https://doi.org/10.1177/1362361315576221

Normand, C. L., Fisher, M. H., Simonato, I., Fecteau, S. M., & Poulin, M. H. (2022). A systematic review of problematic internet use in children, adolescents, and adults with autism spectrum disorder. *Review Journal of Autism and Developmental Disorders, 9*(4), 507–520. https://doi.org/10.1007/s40489-021-00270-x

Raymaker, D. M., McDonald, K. E., Ashkenazy, E., Gerrity, M., Baggs, A. M., Kripke, C., Hourston, S., & Nicolaidis, C. (2017). Barriers to healthcare: Instrument development and comparison between autistic adults and adults with and without other disabilities. *Autism: The International Journal of Research and Practice, 21*(8), 972–984. https://doi.org/10.1177/1362361316661261

Weir, E., Allison, C., & Baron-Cohen, S. (2022). Autistic adults have poorer quality healthcare and worse health based on self-report data. *Molecular Autism, 13*(1), 23. https://doi.org/10.1186/s13 229-022-00501-w

Chapter 2
Autistics in Medical Settings

2.1 Introduction

In this chapter, a summary of the collected literature about autistics in medical settings is presented. This chapter then provides a synopsis about the limitations in the literature reviewed. The final section explains some strategies that can help autistics participate in medical examinations and procedures. The purpose of this section is to answer the research question '*What strategies can be used to help autistics attend dental and medical clinics?*' The purpose of this chapter is to provide the reader with an understanding about some of the common challenges that autistics encounter before and during medical consultations.

2.2 Research Questions About Autistics in Healthcare

2.2.1 What Experiences Have Autistics Had in Medical Clinics?

An examination of the 306 citations collected from the four PubMed searches revealed six studies that answered the research question '*What experiences have autistics had in medical clinics?*' (Brice et al., 2021; Calleja et al., 2020, 2022; Doherty et al., 2022; Mason et al., 2021; Weir et al., 2022). The results from each of these studies will now be explained.

Brice and colleagues (2021) examined what autistics thought about the value and accessibility of modifications to the delivery of mental and physical healthcare. Using mail and online communication methods, over a twelve-month timeframe they gave their survey to autistic adults in the UK who were enrolled with the *Adult Autism Spectrum Cohort—UK*. They discovered that adjustments to the sensory environment, clinical and service factors, and clinician knowledge and communication were

G. Bennett, *Autistic People in Dental and Medical Clinics*, New Perspectives in Behavioral & Health Sciences, https://doi.org/10.1007/978-981-99-2359-5_2

very important for respondents in mental and physical health services (see Table 2.1) (Brice et al., 2021).

Regarding the availability of key adjustments to mental and physical healthcare services to meet the needs of autistic adults, there are many key adjustments that can be made, but they are rarely implemented. For example, respondents claimed that low levels of light were very important in mental health services ($n = 185, 35.2\%$) but were rarely implemented ($n = 101, 40.9\%$) (see Tables 2.1 and 2.2) (Brice et al., 2021).

Based on these results, autistic respondents cited a lack of fundamental modifications in medical clinics. To meet unmet demand and resolve health disparities experienced by autistics in physical and mental healthcare settings, healthcare professionals should change the sensory environment, improve a clinician's knowledge about autism, and improve the communication between autistics and medical professionals (Brice et al., 2021).

Calleja and colleagues (2020) conducted a systematic review to determine the constraints and opportunities for adult autistic patients to receive healthcare. Both quantitative and qualitative studies published between 2003 and 2019 were included in their systematic review. Of the 1290 studies that were originally discovered, 13 were included in their systematic review based on their inclusion and exclusion criteria. Based on their analysis of the collected literature, Calleja and colleagues (2020, p. 7) concluded that:

> This systematic review highlights a global paucity of evidence for autistic adults' access to healthcare. It is vital to support primary healthcare services to better enhance support for autistic adults as this is the first point of call for many individuals. A substantial number of autistic people are transitioning to adult healthcare and will need to access various services for overall wellbeing. Effective communication is the greatest barrier when accessing appropriate services and primary healthcare requires further support as general practitioners play a central role in liaising with services and finding appropriate support for autistic adults.

Unlike the general population, autistic adults typically have greater healthcare demands. However, despite their needs, they still encounter obstacles that prevent them receiving suitable medical treatment. Currently, there is no qualitative study investigating the obstacles to healthcare that impact both the physical and mental health of autistic adults. To address this gap, Calleja and colleagues (2022) performed a qualitative analysis of the reported experiences of healthcare access for autistics ($n = 9$) and the main caregivers for autistic adults ($n = 7$) in Victoria, Australia. They used a three-stage phenomenological approach, which involved a communicative checklist, a health status survey, and face-to-face interviews. They found that healthcare access for autistic adults may be influenced by caregiver behaviours, including support, accountability, and protective factors. As a result of these findings, more study is needed to examine the interrelated factors that affect carers' access to healthcare so that evidence-based treatments may be created to help them in the future.

During 2022, Doherty and colleagues conducted a study to determine the barriers faced by autistics and non-autistics in accessing primary care and the potential impact on their health. They consulted with members of the autistic community at *Autscape*,

Table 2.1 Importance of key adjustments to mental and physical health services to meet the needs of autistic adults

Key adjustment	Mental health services		Physical health services	
	Somewhat important % (N)	Very important % (N)	Somewhat important % (N)	Very important % (N)
Sensory environment				
Change the sensory environment in the building that the appointment will take place in	33.6 (178)	39.4 (209)	31.5 (123)	42.5 (166)
Locations (e.g., waiting rooms) with small numbers of people	30.6 (162)	50.7 (268)	29.4 (116)	52.8 (208)
Locations with low noise levels	28.2 (149)	60.9 (322)	26.4 (104)	61.9 (244)
Locations with low light levels	29.1 (153)	35.2 (185)	31.3 (121)	35.7 (138)
Clinical and service context				
Changing the length of appointments to suit you	33.8 (181)	36.2 (194)	33.9 (134)	44.8 (177)
Offering appointments online or via apps	22.9 (120)	22.9 (120)	18.8 (73)	31.2 (121)
Changing how often you are asked to attend appointments	30.7 (163)	24.5 (130)	28.6 (109)	18.1 (69)
Give information to the clinician pre-appointment so that they can prepare	27.7 (147)	60.6 (322)	32.8 (130)	48.0 (190)
Provide support in relation to attending appointments (e.g., managing fears or uncertainties which might make attending difficult)	27.2 (146)	53.5 (282)	28.0 (109)	50.9 (198)
Appropriate distractions provided while waiting to be seen at appointment (e.g., tablet with headphones)	23.1 (121)	25.2 (132)	24.3 (93)	27.7 (106)
Clinician knowledge and communication				
Clinicians who understand autism	10.7 (57)	87.6 (467)	16.0 (64)	80.5 (322)
Opportunity after the appointment to ask questions about conclusions	31.1 (166)	60.2 (321)	25.4 (100)	64.4 (253)
Appointments at an easily identified and accessible location	19.6 (104)	70.4 (374)	17.1 (70)	71.7 (281)
Appointments with an easily identified and familiar clinician	21.1 (112)	68.9 (365)	19.8 (78)	71.0 (279)
Having a health summary document which can be shared with clinicians (e.g., hospital passport)	28.9 (152)	51.0 (268)	26.0 (100)	48.8 (188)

(continued)

Table 2.1 (continued)

Key adjustment	Mental health services		Physical health services	
	Somewhat important % (N)	Very important % (N)	Somewhat important % (N)	Very important % (N)
A clinician who uses an approach which is informed by what you have said that you prefer (e.g., formal or informal)	31.6 (167)	60.2 (318)	30.6 (118)	50.0 (193)
Identifying reasons that make it difficult to see a clinician or attend an appointment	33.1 (174)	49.5 (260)	29.8 (114)	52.9 (202)
Stand-alone item				
Short waiting times to be seen when you attend appointments	32.5 (168)	55.1 (293)	28.2 (111)	57.8 (227)

Source Brice et al. (2021, p. 7)

an autism-specific conference, and created a self-reported survey consisting of 52 items. The survey was distributed online via social media sites, with a total of 507 autistic adults and 157 non-autistic adults participating. The study found that 80% of autistic respondents and 37% of non-autistic respondents reported difficulties visiting a general practitioner. The most cited obstacles by autistic respondents were deciding if symptoms justified a general practitioner visit (72%), difficulty booking appointments by phone (62%), feeling misunderstood (56%), difficulty speaking with the doctor (53%), and the waiting room environment (51%). Autistic individuals preferred online and text-based appointment scheduling, the ability to email the reason for the visit in advance, first or last appointment times, and a peaceful waiting area. The study also linked self-reported negative health outcomes to obstacles in accessing healthcare. These negative consequences included untreated physical and mental health disorders, missed specialist referrals or screening programmes, needing more extensive treatment or surgery due to late presentation, and untreated potentially life-threatening illnesses. The study found no significant differences between formally diagnosed and self-identified autistic individuals in terms of accessing medical appointments. Healthcare professionals should understand the perspectives, communication needs, and sensory sensitivities of autistic patients to reduce healthcare disparities between autistics and non-autistics. Modifications specific to autistics' needs are just as important as ramps are for wheelchair users.

Mason and colleagues (2021) interviewed healthcare professionals (including physicians and nurses) and conducted focus group discussions with autistics. From these consultations, four main themes emerged, which were:

- Seeing the same professional is important for both autistics and clinicians,
- Both clinicians and autistics believe that adjusting healthcare systems is important and often possible,
- Autistics process information differently and may require extra support in appointments, and
- Clinicians are frequently constrained by time limits and/or targets.

Table 2.2 Lack of availability of key adjustments to mental and physical healthcare services to meet the needs of autistic adults

Key adjustment	Mental health services		Physical health services	
	Somewhat important % (N)	Very important % (N)	Somewhat important % (N)	Very important % (N)
Sensory environment				
Change the sensory environment in the building that the appointment will take place in	26.6 (63)	45.6 (108)	23.1 (55)	60.5 (144)
Locations (e.g., waiting rooms) with small numbers of people	22.3 (63)	29.3 (83)	27.0 (72)	49.1 (131)
Locations with low noise levels	26.0 (72)	26.0 (72)	26.8 (73)	42.6 (116)
Locations with low light levels	24.3 (60)	40.9 (101)	30.9 (76)	52.4 (129)
Clinical and service context				
Changing the length of appointments to suit you	23.1 (52)	45.3 (102)	29.3 (68)	41.4 (96)
Offering appointments online or via apps	16.4 (32)	48.2 (94)	17.6 (41)	32.6 (76)
Changing how often you are asked to attend appointments	25.4 (46)	27.6 (50)	23.1 (34)	44.2 (65)
Give information to the clinician pre-appointment so that they can prepare	22.8 (50)	33.3 (73)	25.1 (56)	41.3 (92)
Provide support in relation to attending appointments (e.g., managing fears or uncertainties which might make attending difficult)	21.7 (51)	40.4 (95)	30.7 (67)	45.9 (100)
Appropriate distractions provided while waiting to be seen at appointment (e.g., tablet with headphones)	15.7 (36)	63.3 (145)	18.3 (38)	66.3 (138)
Clinician knowledge and communication				
Clinicians who understand autism	40.5 (105)	31.3 (81)	36.1 (84)	36.9 (86)
Opportunity after the appointment to ask questions about conclusions	23.9 (63)	18.9 (50)	20.2 (52)	26.8 (69)
Appointments at an easily identified and accessible location	15.3 (47)	10.1 (31)	12.0 (55)	13.0 (38)
Appointments with an easily identified and familiar clinician	18.2 (52)	13.0 (37)	25.3 (73)	16.1 (47)

(continued)

Table 2.2 (continued)

Key adjustment	Mental health services		Physical health services	
	Somewhat important % (N)	Very important % (N)	Somewhat important % (N)	Very important % (N)
Having a health summary document which can be shared with clinicians (e.g., hospital passport)	17.7 (34)	52.1 (100)	17.9 (33)	63.6 (117)
A clinician who uses an approach which is informed by what you have said that you prefer (e.g., formal or informal)	27.9 (70)	23.5 (59)	20.8 (45)	42.1 (91)
Identifying reasons that make it difficult to see a clinician or attend an appointment	25.9 (55)	34.0 (72)	26.3 (52)	46.5 (92)
Stand-alone item				
Short waiting times to be seen when you attend appointments	25.1 (72)	27.2 (78)	33.9 (97)	35.7 (102)

Source Brice et al. (2021, p. 8)

Weir and colleagues (2022) distributed an anonymous, cross-sectional, self-reported questionnaire to 4158 people. The survey collected data about the incidence of chronic diseases, healthcare quality, disparities in overall health inequality scores, and the influence of the coronavirus pandemic on healthcare quality. Fisher's exact test, binomial logistic regression, and predictive machine learning methods were utilised as needed. The sample consisted of 2649 respondents ($n = 1285$ autistics), who ranged in age from 16 to 96 years. Across 50 out of 51 items, autistics reported poorer outcomes compared to non-autistics. Specifically, they reported poorer access to healthcare, more communication problems, more anxiety, sensory sensitivities, system-level issues, and meltdowns than non-autistic adults. Autistic respondents were also more likely than non-autistic respondents to have chronic health issues. Autistic respondents also got somewhat lower-quality healthcare than non-autistic respondents during both the pandemic and the pre-pandemic periods (see Tables 2.3 and 2.4).

2.2.2 What Experiences Have Doctors Had with Treating Autistics?

In response to the question '*What experience have doctors had with treating autistics?*' searches of PubMed revealed two studies that addressed this question (Mason et al., 2021; Morris et al., 2019). Mason and colleagues (2021) conducted interviews with healthcare professionals (including physicians and nurses) and held discussion groups with autistics. Their findings highlighted several key points: seeing the same

Table 2.3 Self-reported lower-quality healthcare experiences for autistic adults compared to non-autistic adults

	Autistic N (%)	Non-autistic N (%)	Unadjusted model OR (95% CI)	p-value	Adjusted model[a] OR (95% CI)	p-value
Able to see healthcare professionals as often as they would like	693 (54.14)	1041 (76.38)	0.365 (0.308, 0.433)	$<2.22 \times 10^{-16}$	0.409 (0.343, 0.487)	$<2.22 \times 10^{-16}$
Has health insurance or is part of a national healthcare programme (e.g., NHS, Medicare, Medicaid, etc.)	991 (78.78)	1095 (82.89)	0.766 (0.626, 0.937)	7.97×10^{-3}	1.026 (0.824, 1.277)	0.818
Sensory experience						
Reported at least one sensory difference (hyper- or hyposensitivity)	1199 (93.31)	609 (44.65)	17.263 (13.494, 22.298)	$<2.22 \times 10^{-16}$	17.984 (13.970, 23.152)	$<2.22 \times 10^{-16}$
I am able to describe how my symptoms feel in my body	707 (55.58)	1174 (87.35)	0.181 (0.148, 0.221)	$<2.22 \times 10^{-16}$	0.187 (0.152, 0.230)	$<2.22 \times 10^{-16}$
I am able to describe how bad my pain feels	650 (51.06)	1129 (84.00)	0.199 (0.165, 0.239)	$<2.22 \times 10^{-16}$	0.193 (0.158, 0.234)	$<2.22 \times 10^{-16}$
I am able to describe my sensory processing differences to healthcare professionals	496 (41.96)	355 (59.97)	0.483 (0.393, 0.593)	1.00×10^{-12}	0.480 (0.388, 0.594)	2.11×10^{-11}
The sensory environment of the waiting room is more overwhelming than other environments	896 (70.44)	420 (31.37)	5.211 (4.398, 6.183)	$<2.22 \times 10^{-16}$	5.253 (4.404, 6.266)	$<2.22 \times 10^{-16}$
The sensory environment of the office is more overwhelming than other environments	745 (58.66)	343 (25.56)	4.131 (3.489, 4.896)	$<2.22 \times 10^{-16}$	4.202 (3.524, 5.011)	$<2.22 \times 10^{-16}$

(continued)

Table 2.3 (continued)

	Autistic N (%)	Non-autistic N (%)	Unadjusted model		Adjusted model[a]	
			OR (95% CI)	p-value	OR (95% CI)	p-value
My senses frequently overwhelm me so that I have trouble focusing on conversations with healthcare professionals	801 (62.97)	240 (17.87)	7.809 (6.503, 9.400)	$<2.22 \times 10^{-16}$	7.587 (6.267, 9.185)	$<2.22 \times 10^{-16}$
Communication						
I am usually able to explain what my symptoms are	848 (66.93)	1213 (91.27)	0.194 (0.153, 0.243)	$<2.22 \times 10^{-16}$	0.202 (0.159, 0.256)	$<2.22 \times 10^{-16}$
I usually understand what my healthcare professional means when they discuss my health	957 (75.47)	1251 (94.20)	0.190 (0.144, 0.248)	$<2.22 \times 10^{-16}$	0.198 (0.150, 0.261)	$<2.22 \times 10^{-16}$
I do not usually ask all the questions I would like to about my health	983 (77.71)	745 (56.31)	2.703 (2.271, 3.223)	$<2.22 \times 10^{-16}$	2.503 (2.089, 2.999)	$<2.22 \times 10^{-16}$
I can bring up a health concern even if my healthcare professional doesn't ask about it	704 (55.65)	1019 (76.96)	0.376 (0.316, 0.446)	$<2.22 \times 10^{-16}$	0.365 (0.304, 0.439)	$<2.22 \times 10^{-16}$
I know what is expected of me when I go to see my healthcare professional	665 (52.45)	1099 (82.82)	0.229 (0.190, 0.275)	$<2.22 \times 10^{-16}$	0.217 (0.179, 0.264)	$<2.22 \times 10^{-16}$
Anxiety						
The idea of going to see a healthcare professional makes me feel anxious	1044 (82.79)	813 (61.73)	2.981 (2.473, 3.602)	$<2.22 \times 10^{-16}$	2.797 (2.308, 3.390)	$<2.22 \times 10^{-16}$

(continued)

Table 2.3 (continued)

	Autistic N (%)	Non-autistic N (%)	Unadjusted model		Adjusted model[a]	
			OR (95% CI)	p-value	OR (95% CI)	p-value
The environment of the waiting room or office makes me feel anxious	1003 (79.67)	602 (45.75)	4.644 (3.887, 5.559)	$<2.22 \times 10^{-16}$	4.509 (3.751, 5.421)	$<2.22 \times 10^{-16}$
I feel anxious when I see a different healthcare professional to whom I expect	1053 (83.70)	595 (45.28)	6.202 (5.140, 7.505)	$<2.22 \times 10^{-16}$	6.111 (5.036, 7.414)	$<2.22 \times 10^{-16}$
The process of setting up an appointment makes me anxious	1053 (83.70)	715 (54.37)	4.308 (3.570, 5.212)	$<2.22 \times 10^{-16}$	4.500 (3.700, 5.475)	$<2.22 \times 10^{-16}$
The process of picking up a prescription makes me anxious	716 (57.05)	320 (24.37)	4.119 (3.471, 4.897)	$<2.22 \times 10^{-16}$	4.084 (3.410, 4.892)	$<2.22 \times 10^{-16}$
I frequently leave my healthcare professional's office feeling as though I did not receive any help at all	786 (62.43)	428 (32.55)	3.442 (2.918, 4.064)	$<2.22 \times 10^{-16}$	3.233 (2.729, 3.830)	$<2.22 \times 10^{-16}$
Access and advocacy						
Chosen not to go in to see a healthcare professional	996 (79.30)	850 (65.69)	2.000 (1.668, 2.402)	1.44×10^{-14}	2.145 (1.777, 2.590)	3.11×10^{-15}
I know who to contact if I have a healthcare concern	951 (75.84)	1120 (86.49)	0.491 (0.397, 0.605)	5.69×10^{-12}	0.449 (0.359, 0.563)	4.43×10^{-12}
If I need to go see a healthcare professional, I am able to get there	1017 (81.30)	1215 (93.82)	0.286 (0.216, 0.376)	$<2.22 \times 10^{-16}$	0.301 (0.225, 0.401)	4.44×10^{-16}
I usually bring someone along to help support me in my appointments	432 (34.45)	267 (20.65)	2.019 (1.684, 2.424)	6.12×10^{-15}	2.296 (1.874, 2.813)	1.55×10^{-15}

(continued)

Table 2.3 (continued)

	Autistic N (%)	Non-autistic N (%)	Unadjusted model		Adjusted model[a]	
			OR (95% CI)	p-value	OR (95% CI)	p-value
If I need to go to the pharmacy, I am able to get there	1101 (87.87)	1252 (96.75)	0.243 (0.167, 0.348)	$<2.22 \times 10^{-16}$	0.294 (0.203, 0.425)	9.67×10^{-11}
I am able to follow a procedure for next steps if asked (e.g., I will attend follow-up appointments, annual check-ups if applicable, etc.)	1009 (80.59)	1188 (91.88)	0.367 (0.285, 0.471)	$<2.22 \times 10^{-16}$	0.348 (0.268, 0.452)	4.22×10^{-15}
I am able to make appointments for myself	1022 (81.56)	1188 (92.09)	0.380 (0.294, 0.489)	2.54×10^{-15}	0.334 (0.252, 0.443)	2.75×10^{-14}
I will wait until it is an emergency before I go to see a healthcare professional	815 (64.99)	673 (52.09)	1.707 (1.451, 2.009)	4.02×10^{-11}	1.619 (1.369, 1.915)	2.09×10^{-8}
System problems						
In most appointments, I have enough time to discuss my concerns with healthcare professionals	515 (41.47)	880 (69.79)	0.307 (0.259, 0.363)	$<2.22 \times 10^{-16}$	0.337 (0.284, 0.401)	$<2.22 \times 10^{-16}$
If I need to go to see a specialist for a healthcare concern, I am able to do so	762 (61.55)	1011 (80.17)	0.396 (0.329, 0.476)	$<2.22 \times 10^{-16}$	0.450 (0.372, 0.545)	4.44×10^{-16}
I often choose not to go to the doctor with concerns if I need to see a specialist because I know that it will take my many appointments before I can see the specialist	702 (56.57)	494 (39.24)	2.016 (1.714, 2.373)	$<2.22 \times 10^{-16}$	1.923 (1.625, 2.277)	4.13×10^{-14}

(continued)

Table 2.3 (continued)

	Autistic N (%)	Non-autistic N (%)	Unadjusted model OR (95% CI)	p-value	Adjusted model[a] OR (95% CI)	p-value
I usually leave my appointments knowing what the next steps are (i.e., follow-up appointments, medications, etc.)	839 (67.66)	1052 (83.76)	0.406 (0.333, 0.493)	$<2.22 \times 10^{-16}$	0.423 (0.345, 0.519)	$<2.22 \times 10^{-16}$
I am provided with appropriate support after I receive a diagnosis of any kind (i.e., anything from infections to chronic conditions)	474 (38.23)	920 (73.25)	0.226 (0.190, 0.269)	$<2.22 \times 10^{-16}$	0.249 (0.209, 0.297)	$<2.22 \times 10^{-16}$
Triggers for a shutdown						
The idea of going to see a healthcare professional	498 (40.65)	138 (11.06)	5.506 (4.446, 6.850)	$<2.22 \times 10^{-16}$	5.623 (4.497, 7.029)	$<2.22 \times 10^{-16}$
Setting up an appointment to see a healthcare professional	470 (38.37)	129 (10.50)	5.305 (4.260, 6.638)	$<2.22 \times 10^{-16}$	5.534 (4.397, 6.963)	$<2.22 \times 10^{-16}$
Sensory environment of the waiting room	538 (43.95)	134 (10.84)	6.445 (5.196, 8.032)	$<2.22 \times 10^{-16}$	6.249 (5.002, 7.808)	$<2.22 \times 10^{-16}$
Sensory environment of the office	457 (37.49)	98 (7.96)	6.934 (5.453, 8.885)	$<2.22 \times 10^{-16}$	6.659 (5.194, 8.538)	$<2.22 \times 10^{-16}$
Seeing a different healthcare professional to whom you expect	467 (38.15)	94 (7.62)	7.475 (5.861, 9.611)	$<2.22 \times 10^{-16}$	7.378 (5.734, 9.493)	$<2.22 \times 10^{-16}$
Talking to a healthcare professional	504 (41.14)	130 (10.53)	5.937 (4.775, 7.419)	$<2.22 \times 10^{-16}$	6.001 (4.777, 7.537)	$<2.22 \times 10^{-16}$
Picking up a prescription	204 (16.68)	46 (3.74)	5.145 (3.676, 7.329)	$<2.22 \times 10^{-16}$	5.076 (3.579, 7.201)	$<2.22 \times 10^{-16}$
Having to see many healthcare professionals before being able to talk to a specialist	510 (41.53)	148 (11.98)	5.213 (4.229, 6.453)	$<2.22 \times 10^{-16}$	4.949 (3.987, 6.143)	$<2.22 \times 10^{-16}$

(continued)

Table 2.3 (continued)

	Autistic N (%)	Non-autistic N (%)	Unadjusted model		Adjusted model[a]	
			OR (95% CI)	p-value	OR (95% CI)	p-value
After a diagnosis of any kind due to lack of follow-up or support	589 (48.52)	179 (14.55)	5.529 (4.537, 6.758)	$<2.22 \times 10^{-16}$	5.405 (4.402, 6.636)	$<2.22 \times 10^{-16}$
Triggers for a meltdown						
The idea of going to see a healthcare professional	209 (17.06)	55 (4.41)	4.460 (3.257, 6.190)	$<2.22 \times 10^{-16}$	4.372 (3.160, 6.050)	$<2.22 \times 10^{-16}$
Setting up an appointment to see a healthcare professional	194 (15.84)	49 (3.99)	4.529 (3.255, 6.401)	$<2.22 \times 10^{-16}$	4.212 (2.998, 5.919)	2.22×10^{-16}
Sensory environment of the waiting room	218 (17.81)	39 (3.16)	6.648 (4.655, 9.703)	$<2.22 \times 10^{-16}$	6.178 (4.298, 8.880)	$<2.22 \times 10^{-16}$
Sensory environment of the office	160 (13.13)	27 (2.19)	6.738 (4.419, 10.634)	$<2.22 \times 10^{-16}$	5.946 (3.874, 9.128)	4.44×10^{-16}
Seeing a different healthcare professional to whom you expect	215 (17.57)	38 (3.08)	6.701 (4.676, 9.828)	$<2.22 \times 10^{-16}$	6.078 (4.212, 8.771)	$<2.22 \times 10^{-16}$
Talking to a healthcare professional	198 (16.16)	42 (3.40)	5.473 (3.861, 7.913)	$<2.22 \times 10^{-16}$	5.299 (3.712, 7.565)	$<2.22 \times 10^{-16}$
Picking up a prescription	116 (9.49)	20 (1.63)	6.330 (3.884, 10.822)	$<2.22 \times 10^{-16}$	5.158 (3.143, 8.466)	1.01×10^{-10}
Having to see many healthcare professionals before being able to talk to a specialist	317 (25.81)	84 (6.80)	4.765 (3.674, 6.232)	$<2.22 \times 10^{-16}$	4.604 (3.519, 6.025)	$<2.22 \times 10^{-16}$
After a diagnosis of any kind due to lack of follow-up or support	394 (32.46)	110 (8.94)	4.889 (3.870, 6.212)	$<2.22 \times 10^{-16}$	4.858 (3.810, 6.195)	$<2.22 \times 10^{-16}$

[a]Binomial Logistic Regression adjusting for age, ethnicity, education, and country of residence

Notes OR odds ratio, *95% CI* 95% confidence interval, *Sig.* significance level

Source Weir et al. (2022, pp. 11–13)

Table 2.4 Autistic adults report lower-quality healthcare than non-autistic peers both before and during the COVID-19 pandemic

	Autistic group N (%)	Control group N (%)	Odds ratio (95% CI)	p-value	Sig.
Pre-Pandemic					
I understood the questions my healthcare professional asked	777 (88.60)	700 (96.82)	0.256 (0.153, 0.411)	2.04×10^{-10}	***
The healthcare professional gave me enough time	630 (71.84)	617 (85.34)	0.438 (0.337, 0.568)	6.97×10^{-11}	***
The healthcare professional understood me when I described my symptoms	616 (70.24)	628 (86.86)	0.357 (0.272, 0.466)	8.39×10^{-16}	***
The healthcare professional attempted to help me with my symptoms	675 (76.97)	629 (87.00)	0.500 (0.378, 0.657)	2.10×10^{-7}	***
I do not think that the healthcare professional cared about my well-being	224 (25.54)	135 (18.67)	1.494 (1.167, 1.917)	0.001	
During Pandemic					
I understood the questions my healthcare professional asked	242 (88.97)	401 (97.09)	0.242 (0.111, 0.498)	2.66×10^{-5}	***
The healthcare professional gave me enough time	200 (73.53)	363 (87.89)	0.383 (0.251, 0.582)	2.23×10^{-6}	***
The healthcare professional understood me when I described my symptoms	196 (72.06)	369 (89.35)	0.308 (0.199, 0.472)	9.96×10^{-9}	***
The healthcare professional attempted to help me with my symptoms	211 (77.57)	377 (91.28)	0.331 (0.205, 0.527)	9.87×10^{-7}	***
I do not think that the healthcare professional cared about my well-being	54 (19.85)	79 (19.13)	1.047 (0.697, 1.566)	0.844	

Notes
95% CI 95% confidence interval, *Sig.* Significance level
p-value: $< 0.001 = *$; $< 0.0001 = **$; $< 0.00001 = ***$
Source Weir et al. (2022, p. 17)

professional is important for both autistics and clinicians; both clinicians and autistics believe that adjusting healthcare is important (and often possible); autistics process information differently and may require extra support in appointments; and clinicians are frequently constrained by time constraints or targets.

There are gaps in our knowledge about the interactions between providers and autistic patients in healthcare settings. To address this lack of knowledge, Morris and colleagues (2019) conducted a scoping study with a focus on exploring the experiences of medical professionals treating autistic patients. After a comprehensive search and examination of the literature, they discovered 27 studies that were of interest. These 27 studies were characterised by six major themes, which were:

1. complexity beyond usual role,
2. limited knowledge and resources,
3. training/prior experience,
4. communication and collaboration,
5. need for information and training, and
6. need for care coordination and systemic changes.

The results of this study have implications for future research and practice, and they should be addressed when considering how to improve research and service provision for autistic patients.

2.2.3   What Experiences Have Parents Had with Their Autistic Child Receiving Medical Care?

Two studies retrieved from the searches of PubMed were judged to answer the research question 'What experiences have parents had with their autistic child receiving medical care?' (Boshoff et al., 2021; Calleja et al., 2022). These studies are now described.

Boshoff and colleagues (2021) conducted a systematic review of qualitative research to present a better understanding of parental experiences of supporting their autistic child to access healthcare services. Their review question was 'How do parents of children with autism describe their experiences of utilising routine healthcare services?' A modified version of the Critical Appraisal Skills Program instrument was used by paired reviewers to independently evaluate 12 papers that had been found after a thorough search and selection procedure. The Joanna Briggs approach for meta-aggregation was used by two reviewers to synthesise the data. The 12 studies that made up this evaluation (which covered the years 2012 to 2020) reflected the opinions of 240 parents. The synthesis showed that typically parents described difficulties accessing and using conventional health treatments for their autistic child owing to a lack of a voice, limited communication, and a lack of understanding from healthcare providers. Their review of the literature adds to our understanding of parents' experiences with healthcare services and will help healthcare professionals re-evaluate their own communication, comprehension, and approach with autistic children and their families. Based on their findings, they proposed that healthcare practitioners should include parents' views in healthcare visits more often. Their insights will aid in the delivery of effective, supportive, and positive healthcare experiences for all parties involved.

Unlike the general population, autistic adults have greater healthcare demands. However, despite their needs, they still encounter obstacles in receiving the right treatment. Currently, there is no qualitative study investigating the obstacles that impact both the physical and mental health of autistic adults. To address this gap, Calleja and colleagues (2022) performed a qualitative analysis of the reported experiences of healthcare access for autistics ($n = 9$) and main caregivers of autistic adults ($n = 7$) in Victoria, Australia. They used a three-staged phenomenological approach, which involved (i) a communicative checklist, (ii) a health status survey, and (iii) face-to-face interviews. Healthcare access for autistic adults may be influenced by caregiver behaviours, including support, accountability, and protective factors. As a result of the findings, further study is needed to examine the interrelated factors that affect carers' access to healthcare so that evidence-based treatments may be created to help caregivers in the future.

2.2.4 What Barriers Prevent Autistics from Receiving Medical Care?

An examination of the 306 citations collected from the four PubMed searches revealed three studies that answered the research question 'What barriers prevent autistics from receiving medical care?' (Mason et al., 2019; Shawahna et al., 2021; Wilson & Peterson, 2018). The results from each of these studies will now be explained.

Mason and colleagues (2019) published a systematic review of articles about the obstacles and enablers that influence access to healthcare for autistic patients. They examined six articles and identified a series of barriers (see Table 2.5) (see Appendix 2.1).

A lack of knowledge about the autism spectrum can be a barrier that prevents autistic patients from receiving suitable medical treatment. Shawahna and colleagues (2021) examined medical students' familiarity, expertise, and confidence in understanding the autism spectrum and autistics. Their multicentre, cross-sectional study was done among medical students at Palestine's three main medical institutions. In addition to sociodemographic and academic information, the questionnaire assessed experience of the autism spectrum (8 items), knowledge about the autism spectrum (12 items), and confidence and readiness to learn about the autism spectrum (5 items). In total, 309 medical students completed the questionnaire, which equated to a response rate of 77.3%. As outlined in the table below, out of the eight indicators of familiarity with the autism spectrum posed the respondents were 'not familiar' with five of these indicators (see Table 2.6) (Shawahna et al., 2021).

Table 2.5 Barriers to healthcare access reported across studies (listed in order of consistency of findings across studies)

Barrier(s)	Studies					
	Nicolaidis et al. (2015)	Dern and Sappok (2016)	Nicolaidis et al. (2016)	Raymaker et al. (2017)	Vogan et al. (2017)	Saqr et al. (2018)
Communication (i.e., atypical communication, literal interpretation, making appointments)	+	+	+	+		+
Sensory sensitivities (including the waiting room, physical examination)	+	+	+	+		+
Challenges with bodily awareness (i.e., difficulty describing pain or symptoms)	+	+	+	+	+	
Providers' degree of flexibility (i.e., allowing written communication, using accessible language, making needed accommodations)	+	+	+	+		+
Slow processing speed (i.e., during social interaction) or executive functioning (i.e., self-regulating medication, missing appointments)	+	+	+	+		
Providers' negative attitudes (i.e., misinterpreting behaviours, communication is not taken seriously)	+		+	+	+	
Availability of supports (both formal and informal; fear of social isolation)	+		+	+	+	

(continued)

Table 2.5 (continued)

Barrier(s)	Studies					
	Nicolaidis et al. (2015)	Dern and Sappok (2016)	Nicolaidis et al. (2016)	Raymaker et al. (2017)	Vogan et al. (2017)	Saqr et al. (2018)
Healthcare system is too complex or inaccessible (including not knowing where to find help)	+		+	+	+	
Emotional (i.e., anxiety or embarrassment)			+	+	+	+
Challenges with organisation (i.e., remembering to take medication, making or attend appointments)	+	+	+	+		
Need for consistency (i.e., seeing the same staff)	+	+	+			
Providers' (lack of) knowledge about autism in adults (including making assumptions about behaviour, or lacking confidence in treating autistic patients)	+		+	+		
Negative experiences with healthcare (including lack of trust in professional help, not including the autistic patient in healthcare discussions)	+			+	+	
Stigma about autism	+		+		+	
Other societal issues that affect health (including socioeconomic factors)	+			+		
Highly variable needs of autistic people			+			+
Distance too far to get help				+	+	
The problem did not seem so serious					+	
Want to handle the problem ourselves [the autistic person]					+	
Too busy/other priorities					+	

(continued)

Table 2.5 (continued)

Barrier(s)	Studies					
	Nicolaidis et al. (2015)	Dern and Sappok (2016)	Nicolaidis et al. (2016)	Raymaker et al. (2017)	Vogan et al. (2017)	Saqr et al. (2018)
Problem was considered temporary					+	
Other people did not want the family to seek help					+	

Notes + Barrier is reported by this study
Source Mason et al. (2019, p. 3394)

Respondents in Shawahna et al.'s (2021) study were also asked twelve true/false/don't know questions about the aetiology, prevalence, and treatment of the autism spectrum. The purpose of these questions was to test their level of accurate knowledge about the autism spectrum. As illustrated in the table below, most respondents answered the questions correctly (see Table 2.7) (Shawahna et al., 2021).

Wilson and Peterson (2018) examined 29 studies that described the experiences in medical care settings from the perspective of autistic patients younger than 18 years of age and their caregivers. Their review of the literature showed that parent-reported problems in parent-provider communication and overwhelming sensory environments hampered the medical treatment that autistic children received.

2.3 Limitations of the Current Research

2.3.1 *Experiences of Autistics in Medical Clinics*

An examination of the citations collected from the four PubMed searches revealed six studies that answered the question '*What experiences have autistics had in medical clinics?*' An inspection of these six studies revealed a series of limitations that can potentially undermine the results. Brice and colleagues (2021) claimed that the insights that they examined were based on the autistic participants' recollections. They did not verify these recollections by asking service providers for their comments. Based on the studies that they examined for their literature review, Calleja and colleagues (2020) concluded that it was difficult to evaluate the effectiveness of enablers to healthcare access for autistic adults because the studies they reviewed had diverse participant numbers and demographics, measurement and analysis tools, and length of data collection. Calleja and colleagues (2022) admitted that their results were based on a small sample size of autistic adults ($n = 9$) and primary caregivers of autistic children ($n = 7$). Consequently, it is not possible to generalise the results discovered to the broader autistic population. Doherty and colleagues (2022)

Table 2.6 Familiarity of the medical students with symptoms, diagnosis, treatment options, and community resources to help autistics and their families

#	Familiarity item	Not familiar at all		Not familiar		Somewhat familiar		Familiar		Completely familiar	
		n	%	n	%	n	%	n	%	n	%
	How would you rate your familiarity with										
1	Different symptoms of ASDs	13	4.2	63	20.4	**167**	**54.0**	53	17.2	13	4.2
2	Different tools used to diagnose ASDs	50	16.2	**142**	**46.0**	93	30.1	18	5.8	6	1.9
3	Different classes of drugs (e.g., antidepressants, antipsychotics, central nervous system stimulants) that can be used in the management of the symptoms of ASDs	38	12.3	107	34.6	**108**	**35.0**	52	16.8	4	1.3
4	Specific behaviours associated with ASDs that drugs seek to alleviate (e.g., self-injury, hyperactivity, and obsessive–compulsive disorder)	24	7.8	68	22.0	**132**	**42.7**	68	22.0	17	5.5
5	Doses of drugs used in the management of symptoms of ASDs	95	30.7	**143**	**46.3**	47	15.2	20	6.5	4	1.3
6	Various side effects produced by drugs used in the management of symptoms of ASDs (e.g., irritation, sedation, and extrapyramidal symptoms)	47	15.2	**131**	**42.4**	92	29.8	34	11.0	5	1.6
7	How to help families sort through information to make informed decisions about their child with ASDs	30	9.7	**121**	**39.2**	111	35.9	42	13.6	5	1.6

(continued)

Table 2.6 (continued)

#	Familiarity item	Not familiar at all		Not familiar		Somewhat familiar		Familiar		Completely familiar	
		n	%	n	%	n	%	n	%	n	%
8	Community resources available in the region that can be used for referral of a child who is exhibiting symptoms commonly associated with ASDs	44	14.2	**125**	**40.5**	100	32.4	33	10.7	7	2.3

Notes Answers with the most responses are **boldface**
Source Shawahna et al. (2021, p. 6)

Table 2.7 Knowledge of the medical students with aetiology, prevalence, and treatment of the autism spectrum

#	Knowledge item	True		False		I don't know		
		n	*%*	*n*	*%*	*n*	*%*	D
1	ASDs are developmental disorders?	**187**	**60.5**	57	18.4	65	21.0	Easy
2	Children with ASDs have impairments in social interaction, communication or language, and behavioural development?	**288**	**93.2**	6	1.9	15	4.9	Very easy
3	ASDs occur more commonly among males than females?	**123**	**39.8**	27	8.7	159	51.5	Difficult
4	ASDs are more prevalent than juvenile diabetes?	**40**	**12.9**	58	18.8	211	68.3	Very difficult
5	ASDs are more prevalent than Down syndrome?	**66**	**21.4**	82	26.5	161	52.1	Difficult
6	ASDs are curable?	45	14.6	**193**	**62.5**	71	23.0	Easy
7	Risperidone and aripiprazole have been approved by the health authorities for the treatment of irritability associated with ASDs?	**53**	**17.2**	13	4.2	243	78.6	Very difficult
8	Vaccines can cause ASDs?	23	7.4	**207**	**67.0**	79	25.6	Easy
9	ASDs exist only in childhood?	59	19.1	**199**	**64.4**	51	16.5	Easy
10	ASDs are caused because of emotionally distant, rejecting parents?	102	33.0	**133**	**43.0**	74	23.9	Moderate
11	Genetic factors play a major role in the aetiology of ASDs?	**219**	**70.9**	31	10.0	59	19.1	Easy
12	ASDs are rare disorder?	37	12.0	**199**	**64.4**	73	23.6	Easy

Notes Correct answers are **boldface**
Source Shawahna et al. (2021, p. 6)

acknowledged that for their study respondents needed to complete a survey and that their survey did not take into consideration potential confounding factors, such as the participant's ethnicity and socioeconomic status. Their sample also contained an overrepresentation of autistic females ($n = 311$, 62%) than autistic males ($n = 99$, 20%). The design of their study resulted in autistic adults who were not capable of completing the survey being excluded and confounding factors not being taken into consideration during data analysis. Mason and colleagues (2021) also disclosed that they did not collect details about the participant's ethnicity, measures of autistic traits, co-occurring conditions (e.g., mental health), or the number of times each participant interacted with health services. This lack of details impacted their ability to analyse the impact of these confounding factors on the health outcomes of autistics. Finally, Weir and colleagues (2022) revealed that their results could not be generalised to the entire autistic population since their survey was only completed by those who were able to complete a survey.

To improve our understanding about the experiences of autistics in medical clinics, there are three design modifications that studies in the future should adopt to address the limitations in the current research. First, researchers should design studies in which they validate the experiences autistics disclose by comparing them against those of their parents and healthcare professionals. This should address the short-coming revealed by Brice and colleagues. Second, Doherty and colleagues, and Mason and colleagues (2021) explained that they did not collect confounding factors from participants, such as the participant's ethnicity and socioeconomic status. This detail should be collected so a more complex analysis of the healthcare situations that autistics have encountered can be conducted. Third, participants in studies by Weir and colleagues and Doherty and colleagues had to complete a survey. This approach excluded those who were unable to complete their survey and, conse-quently, hampered the generalisability of the results created. To ensure that the insights from those unable to complete a survey are collected and examined, studies in the future should give participants other means to explain their experiences in the healthcare system. For example, interviewing participants or allowing them to either write or audio record such experiences.

2.3.2   Experiences Doctors Have Had with Treating Autistics

From the four PubMed searches, two studies were deemed to answer the research question 'What experiences have doctors had with treating autistics?' (Mason et al., 2021; Morris et al., 2019). Within these two studies, the authors explained the limi-tations in their research. Mason and colleagues explained that all clinicians who participated in their study were recruited from the Northeast region of England. Consequently, their insights might not be representative of professionals in other parts of the country. Morris and colleagues explained that of the 27 studies that they reviewed for their literature review, 17 were conducted in the United States. Consequently, the results in these 17 studies may not be applicable in an international context.

To improve our knowledge about the experiences of medical professionals treating autistics, there are two design modifications that studies in the future should adopt. First, medical professionals from a more diverse geographical area should be recruited. This will ensure that the results collected from medical professionals can be generalised. Second, more non-American research about medical professionals treating autistic patients should be published. This will address Morris et al.'s concerns that the results about this topic cannot be applied to those who live outside the United States.

2.3.3   Parental Experiences of Their Autistic Child Receiving Medical Care

In response to the question 'What experiences have parents had with their autistic child receiving medical care?' two studies were identified from the four separate PubMed searches (Boshoff et al., 2021; Calleja et al., 2022). Within these two studies, the authors explained the limitations in their research. Calleja and colleagues (2022) acknowledged that the results in their study were based on a small number of caregivers who support autistic adults ($n = 7$). Thus, the results could not be generalised to the broader population of caregivers of autistic adults. Boshoff and colleagues (2021) claimed that the research that they reviewed was published in English. Thus, findings published in languages other than English were not examined. They also claimed that:

> Due to the limited number of studies identified for inclusion in this review and their varying methodological quality, primary research into the parental experiences is needed to further our understanding of healthcare visits of parents with children with autism. Future studies are recommended that focus on children with more severe levels of autism and with parents across the range of socioeconomic, educational and cultural demographics. (Boshoff et al., 2021, p. 1680)

To enhance our understanding about the experiences of parents supporting their autistic children in healthcare settings, studies in the future should adopt three changes in their design. First, to correct the limitation in Calleja et al.'s (2022) study, the number of parents of autistic children in studies should increase. This expanded sample size can ensure that the results obtained can be generalised to the broader population. Second, researchers should collect more details about the socioeconomic, educational, and cultural demographics about parents supporting their autistic children in healthcare settings. Third, more research that focuses on the experiences of parents supporting children with more severe levels of autism in healthcare should be conducted. By adopting these strategies, the limitations articulated by Boshoff and colleagues would be addressed.

2.3.4 Barriers That Prevent Autistics from Receiving
Medical Care

An examination of the citations retrieved from the four separate searches of PubMed revealed three studies that answered the question '*What barriers prevent autistics from receiving medical care?*' (Mason et al., 2019; Shawahna et al., 2021; Wilson & Peterson, 2018). Within these three studies, the authors explained the limitations in their research. For their scoping review, Mason and colleagues (2019) examined six studies. Consequently, the results from these studies could not be generalised to a broad range of situations. In Shawahna and colleagues study, participants were required to answer a series of multiple-choice questions. Such questions resulted in the survey being biased since respondents could only answer preconceived answers. Another limitation of Shawahna and colleagues' study was that despite medical students being recruited from three major universities in Palestine the sample size was relatively small (i.e., $n = 309$). Finally, Wilson and Peterson (2018) admitted that most of the studies examined for their scoping review were conducted in the United States. Thus, the results were American centric since there was not a lot of international research.

To enhance our understanding about the barriers that autistics encounter when receiving medical care, two changes need to be implemented in research conducted in the future. First, more research about the barriers that prevent autistics from accessing healthcare should be conducted. Such research would improve our ability to generalise the results to different medical settings. Second, more research about the hurdles that autistics encounter when accessing medical care should be conducted in nations other than the United States. This would ensure that the current literature is not American centric and can be applied to other nations.

2.4 Strategies to Assist Autistics in Medical Settings

2.4.1 Explaining the Medical Procedure Before
Its Commencement

Often autistics experience anxiety when they are in situations where they are unsure about the medical procedures that they will undergo. To combat this anxiety, it is recommended that before a medical procedure begins the doctor should clearly and comprehensively explain each individual step involved in the medical procedure. In some situations, visual diagrams may help convey complex medical procedures with lucidity.

2.4.2 Removing Sensory Sensitivities from the Clinical Environment

Some autistics have sensory sensitivities that might have an impact on their ability to tolerate medical encounters. Most autistic respondents who participated in Brice et al.'s (2021) study reported that they preferred clinical environments that had low noise levels ($n = 224$, 61.9%). This point was also echoed in Weir et al.'s (2022) study, with more autistic participants supporting the claim that '*the sensory environment of the waiting room is more overwhelming than other environments*' (autistic respondents $n = 896$, 70.44%; non-autistic respondents $n = 420$, 31.37%). To subdue the sensory discomfort that autistic patients experience in clinical environments, doctors and practice managers should ask autistic patients about their sensory experiences in the clinic. For their study, Weir and colleagues (2022) designed a healthcare satisfaction survey which has been adapted to suit the needs of clinics (see Appendix 2.2).

2.4.3 Giving Autistic Patients a Form That They Can Use to Explain Their Healthcare Needs

Some autistic patients have encountered difficulties while explaining to doctors their medical problems. In Weir et al.'s (2022) study, 504 (41.14%) autistic respondents claimed that talking to a healthcare professional was a trigger for a shutdown while 198 (16.16%) autistic respondents claimed that it was a trigger for a meltdown. In Doherty et al.'s (2022) study, 53% of autistic respondents claimed that they had trouble expressing their medical concerns to a doctor. To help overcome this barrier, the *National Autistic Society* has created the *My Health Passport*, a form that some autistics can complete to inform the doctor about their medical concerns. Appendix 2.3 is a modified version of this form that doctors can use in their medical clinics. The usage of a *My Health Passport* has been endorsed by autistics. In Brice et al.'s (2021) study, 188 autistics (48.8%) explained that it was '*very important*' that they have a health summary document that they can share with clinicians and 100 autistics (26%) said that such a summary document was '*somewhat important*' in physical health services.

2.4.4 Educating Medical Students About Autism

Medical students have explained that while studying in medical school they did not receive adequate training about the autism spectrum or how to support autistic patients (Austriaco et al., 2019; Clarke & Fung, 2022; Low & Zailan, 2016). To mitigate the difficulties that future generations of medical students will encounter while trying to support autistic patients, it is vital that universities update their medical curriculums so that medical students acquire a proficient level of knowledge about autism and how to support autistics. Furthermore, such education should be respectful of autistics so that situations of embarrassment, as illustrated below, are avoided:

> … one day a senior academic, who I had been working with for several years, asked me to participate in his talk. I stood on the stage as I was introduced to the packed conference: "This is Cos, an autistic adult." So there I was, a woman in late middle age, fully equipped with white hair and breasts; yet apparently this needed stating, out loud, to my face, in front of an audience. I was being shown off as a specimen and I was mortified. … Remember those Victorian etchings of public lectures, with all the toffs in starched collars and monocles and the solitary wild haired, drug eyed mute, led on in a canvas shift? Yup—it felt just like that. (Michael, 2021, p. 118)

2.5 Conclusion

This chapter presented a summary of the literature about autistics in medical settings that was collected from the four searches of PubMed. By classifying the literature, each research question was answered. This chapter then provided a summary about the limitations in the literature reviewed. The final section explained some strategies that can help autistics have uneventful experiences while undergoing medical examinations and procedures. This section answered the research question '*What strategies can be used to help autistics attend dental and medical clinics?*' Overall, the purpose of this chapter was to provide the reader with an understanding about some of the common challenges that autistics encounter before and during medical consultations.

References

Austriaco, K., Aban, I., Willig, J., & Kong, M. (2019). Contemporary trainee knowledge of autism: How prepared are our future providers? *Frontiers in Pediatrics, 7*, 165. https://doi.org/10.3389/fped.2019.00165

Boshoff, K., Bowen-Salter, H., Gibbs, D., Phillips, R. L., Porter, L., & Wiles, L. (2021). A meta-synthesis of how parents of children with autism describe their experience of accessing and using routine healthcare services for their children. *Health & Social Care in the Community, 29*(6), 1668–1682. https://doi.org/10.1111/hsc.13369

Brice, S., Rodgers, J., Ingham, B., Mason, D., Wilson, C., Freeston, M., Le Couteur, A., & Parr, J. R. (2021). The importance and availability of adjustments to improve access for autistic adults who need mental and physical healthcare: Findings from UK surveys. *BMJ Open, 11*(3), e043336. https://doi.org/10.1136/bmjopen-2020-043336

Calleja, S., Islam, F. M. A., Kingsley, J., & McDonald, R. (2020). Healthcare access for autistic adults: A systematic review. *Medicine, 99*(29), e20899. https://doi.org/10.1097/MD.0000000000020899

Calleja, S., Kingsley, J., Amirul Islam, F. M., & McDonald, R. (2022). Barriers to accessing healthcare: Perspectives from autistic adults and carers. *Qualitative Health Research, 32*(2), 267–278. https://doi.org/10.1177/10497323211050362

Clarke, L., & Fung, L. K. (2022). The impact of autism-related training programs on physician knowledge, self-efficacy, and practice behavior: A systematic review. *Autism: The International Journal of Research and Practice, 26*(7), 1626–1640. https://doi.org/10.1177/136236132211 02016

Dern, S., & Sappok, T. (2016). Barriers to healthcare for people on the autism spectrum. *Advances in Autism, 2*(1), 2–11. https://doi.org/10.1108/AIA-10-2015-0020

Doherty, M., Neilson, S., O'Sullivan, J., Carravallah, L., Johnson, M., Cullen, W., & Shaw, S. C. K. (2022). Barriers to healthcare and self-reported adverse outcomes for autistic adults: A cross-sectional study. *BMJ Open, 12*(2), e056904. https://doi.org/10.1136/bmjopen-2021-056904

Low, H. M., & Zailan, F. (2016). Medical students' perceptions, awareness, societal attitudes and knowledge of autism spectrum disorder: An exploratory study in Malaysia. *International Journal of Developmental Disabilities, 64*(2), 86–95. https://doi.org/10.1080/20473869.2016.1264663

Mason, D., Ingham, B., Birtles, H., Michael, C., Scarlett, C., James, I. A., Brown, T., Woodbury-Smith, M., Wilson, C., Finch, T., & Parr, J. R. (2021). How to improve healthcare for autistic people: A qualitative study of the views of autistic people and clinicians. *Autism: The International Journal of Research and Practice, 25*(3), 774–785. https://doi.org/10.1177/136236132 1993709

Mason, D., Ingham, B., Urbanowicz, A., Michael, C., Birtles, H., Woodbury-Smith, M., Brown, T., James, I., Scarlett, C., Nicolaidis, C., & Parr, J. R. (2019). A systematic review of what barriers and facilitators prevent and enable physical healthcare services access for autistic adults. *Journal of Autism and Developmental Disorders, 49*(8), 3387–3400. https://doi.org/10.1007/s10 803-019-04049-2

Michael, C. (2021). Is being othered a co-occurring condition of autism? *Autism in Adulthood, 3*(2), 118–119. https://doi.org/10.1089/aut.2021.0019

Morris, R., Greenblatt, A., & Saini, M. (2019). Healthcare providers' experiences with autism: A scoping review. *Journal of Autism and Developmental Disorders, 49*(6), 2374–2388. https://doi. org/10.1007/s10803-019-03912-6

Nicolaidis, C., Raymaker, D. M., Ashkenazy, E., McDonald, K. E., Dern, S., Baggs, A. E., Kapp, S. K., Weiner, M., & Boisclair, W. C. (2015). "Respect the way I need to communicate with you": Healthcare experiences of adults on the autism spectrum. *Autism: The International Journal of Research and Practice, 19*(7), 824–831. https://doi.org/10.1177/1362361315576221

Nicolaidis, C., Raymaker, D., McDonald, K., Kapp, S., Weiner, M., Ashkenazy, E., Gerrity, M., Kripke, C., Platt, L., & Baggs, A. (2016). The development and evaluation of an online healthcare toolkit for autistic adults and their primary care providers. *Journal of General Internal Medicine, 31*(10), 1180–1189. https://doi.org/10.1007/s11606-016-3763-6

Raymaker, D. M., McDonald, K. E., Ashkenazy, E., Gerrity, M., Baggs, A. M., Kripke, C., Hourston, S., & Nicolaidis, C. (2017). Barriers to healthcare: Instrument development and comparison between autistic adults and adults with and without other disabilities. *Autism: The International Journal of Research and Practice, 21*(8), 972–984. https://doi.org/10.1177/1362361316661261

Saqr, Y., Braun, E., Porter, K., Barnette, D., & Hanks, C. (2018). Addressing medical needs of adolescents and adults with autism spectrum disorders in a primary care setting. *Autism: The International Journal of Research and Practice, 22*(1), 51–61. https://doi.org/10.1177/136236 1317709970

Shawahna, R., Jaber, M., Yahya, N., Jawadeh, F., & Rawajbeh, S. (2021). Are medical students in Palestine adequately trained to care for individuals with autism spectrum disorders? A multi-center cross-sectional study of their familiarity, knowledge, confidence, and willingness to learn. *BMC Medical Education, 21*(1), 424. https://doi.org/10.1186/s12909-021-02865-8

Vogan, V., Lake, J. K., Tint, A., Weiss, J. A., & Lunsky, Y. (2017). Tracking health care service use and the experiences of adults with autism spectrum disorder without intellectual disability: A longitudinal study of service rates, barriers and satisfaction. *Disability and Health Journal, 10*(2), 264–270. https://doi.org/10.1016/j.dhjo.2016.11.002

Weir, E., Allison, C., & Baron-Cohen, S. (2022). Autistic adults have poorer quality healthcare and worse health based on self-report data. *Molecular Autism, 13*(1), 23. https://doi.org/10.1186/s13 229-022-00501-w

Wilson, S. A., & Peterson, C. C. (2018). Medical care experiences of children with autism and their parents: A scoping review. *Child: Care, Health and Development, 44*(6), 807–817. https://doi. org/10.1111/cch.12611

Chapter 3
Autistics in Dental Clinics

3.1 Introduction

This chapter begins with a summary of the literature that answers the research questions about autistics in dental settings. This is followed by a selection that summarises the limitations in the reviewed literature. The final section explains some strategies that can help autistics participate in dental examinations and procedures. The purpose of this section is to answer the research question '*What strategies can be used to help autistics attend dental and medical clinics?*' The contents in this chapter will help the reader understand some of the challenges that autistics encounter before and during dental examinations.

3.2 Autistics in Dental Clinics

3.2.1 *What Experiences Have Autistics Had in Dental Clinics?*

In response to the question '*What experiences have autistics had in dental clinics?*' the four distinct searches of PubMed revealed two studies that addressed this question (McMillion et al., 2021; Mirsky et al., 2021).

Studies have demonstrated that sensory processing, anxiety, and communication problems make it difficult for autistic adults to obtain dental treatment. It is unknown, though, if autistic adults in the UK encountered similar obstacles to receiving dental treatment. To determine if autistic adults had more bad experiences than non-autistic adults, McMillion and colleagues (2021) administered a mixed-methods survey to self-identified autistic ($n = 37$) and non-autistic ($n = 43$) adults. Several questions were designed to obtain information about the dental environment, patient-practitioner communication, anxiety, and satisfaction. Open questions regarding how to make the dental experience better for autistics, what worked well, and dental issues unique to autism were posed to autistics. Thematic analysis was used to examine the responses. Overall, the findings showed that autistics in the UK have more unpleasant dental encounters than non-autistic adults. Particularly, autistics had difficulties with the sensory environment, dental professionals, fear, discomfort, and challenges with disclosing that they are autistic. Autistic respondents suggested adjusting the sensory environment, strategies to be more prepared, and lengthier appointments. This study emphasised the significance of dentists working with autistics to optimise the quality of care and outcomes while providing best-practice techniques for working with autistic patients.

Autistics deserve to be treated by healthcare professionals, such as dentists, that understand and are attentive to their sensitivities and requirements. The objective of Mirsky et al.'s (2021) study was to learn more about the dental experiences and requirements of young autistics. Purposive and snowball sampling approaches were used to recruit young autistics for their qualitative descriptive study. Semi-structured, open-ended interviews were conducted and audio recorded. To preserve the participant's confidentiality, pseudonyms were used. At the time of data collection, interviews were transcribed and the data was processed concurrently. To generate common categories, open and axial coding techniques were used. Triangulation and member verification were used to ensure validity. From the interviews, five conceptual themes emerged, which were:

1. emotional experiences related to oral care visits (see Table 3.1),
2. likes and dislikes related to oral healthcare delivery (see Table 3.2),
3. communication techniques (see Table 3.3),
4. oral self-care recommendations likes and dislikes (see Table 3.4), and
5. sensory challenges during oral healthcare (see Table 3.5).

Table 3.1 Emotional experiences about oral care visits

Emotional experience	Quote
Positive emotions or feelings	'I'm pretty happy when I visit there. There's a slight bit of nervousness, but it's nothing to make me panic or anything like that. I'm generally calm. I'm still pretty happy when I visit the hygienist, but the only difference is that there's zero nervousness when it comes to dental hygienists. That's way more relaxed. I was a weird kid. I loved the dentist. I'm generally very calm, very happy going. - Kevin'
Neutral emotions or feelings	'I feel all right. I just feel like it's what has to be done. They're just checking me out, not doing anything bad. And so I just follow it. Because I can't do this by myself. I'm sure my teeth are okay but there's always professionals doing it, making sure I don't get cavities and they point out what I may need some help with. - Elaine'
	'I feel, to be honest, pretty neutral when I go. It's like another thing in my life to do. - Evans'
Negative emotions or feelings	'I don't know if they're going to hurt me or if they're not going to hurt me and I have to play it in my head that nothing's going to happen, but there's always that fear that's there. - Rose'

Table 3.2 Likes and dislikes related to oral healthcare delivery

Emotional experience	Quote
Dental hygiene care Liked	*'The thing I like the most is that once it's done your teeth are clean and you know what you're supposed to do to improve if you've been lacking in a certain area. Also, the people there are always nice. They give you a bag of stuff. … - Ethan'*
Dental hygiene care Disliked	*'Those scrapers, those small metal hooks that scrape the teeth for any plaque. It kind of gives me goosebumps, if it gets to a bad area almost close to my gums. … - Elaine'*
Dental treatment Liked	*'My dentist that I go to is really kind. He really knows how to take care of me and make me feel comfortable. He does give me support and encouragement to keep up the good work on my brushing. I like him. I just like his smile. He has a pretty jovial attitude. He's very kind, very friendly and the people that work with him are very nice as well. - Quinn'*
Dental treatment Disliked	*'In the moment I'm just thinking, okay when the dentist comes I have no idea what they're going to do. The part I hate the most is not when the dentist comes, it's everything before that, not knowing what's going to happen. - Sophia'*

3.2.2 What Experiences Have Dentists Had with Treating Autistics?

Two studies retrieved from the four distinct searches of PubMed were judged to answer the research question *'What experiences have dentists had with treating autistics?'* (Eades et al., 2019; McMillion et al., 2022).

The experiences of dental professionals in treating autistic patients in the UK have not been extensively studied. Eades and colleagues (2019) investigated dental professionals' knowledge of autism, their confidence in treating autistic patients, and the factors that affect their confidence. An online survey was conducted among 482 dental professionals in the UK. The results indicate that more than half of the respondents have not received formal autism training, but their average knowledge level is good. However, their confidence levels in treating autistic patients were only moderate. Respondents often cited a lack of resources to implement support strategies, despite understanding the additional needs of autistic patients. Nevertheless, most respondents were positive about making the necessary modifications to support their autistic patients. This study highlights the need for better training initiatives to improve dental professionals' confidence and ability to meet the needs of autistic patients.

Previous research has shown that autistics often have difficulty receiving dental treatment due to both autism-specific issues and practitioners' views about autism. There is, however, a dearth of research about dentists' interactions with their autistic patients. The purpose of McMillion et al.'s (2022) study was to examine the methods dental practitioners in the UK employ while treating autistic patients. For their study, 16 dental professionals from a range of specialised fields, including special care, paediatrics, and orthodontics, participated. They were asked to comprehensively

Table 3.3 Communication techniques

Emotional experience	Quote
Positive communication experiences	'I talk to them like they're another person. Usually, I'm not really the best at starting conversations. They meet me, they welcome me. We have a little conversation. Like, how are you doing? Hi, how's your day been? And then we get into the process of cleaning up our teeth. Maybe if I don't feel comfortable with something they're doing within my mouth, I'll make a noise or I'll ask for something, they'll usually provide it. If something feels painful, they'll try and lighten it a bit, so that there's not as much pressure being put on it, so that it doesn't hurt as much. - Evans'
Negative communication experiences	'If I didn't do a good job cleaning my teeth, [I would be] scolded by the dentist or dental hygienist afterwards. - Bob'
Positive non-verbal communication	'My current dentist, who I've seen a couple times, I really like. She's the only one I've ever met who takes the conversations that happen behind you and moves them in front of you. She's talking with the dental hygienist, she's getting everything ready within my field of vision, and she's explaining things to me. She's doing the things that I appreciate about my dental hygienist that I think come from having more time, not being as rushed. I really like when she engages me instead of just opening my mouth and sticking stuff in there. - Sophia'
Negative non-verbal communication	'I don't like that I can't read their faces as well because they have a mask on, or they're somewhere where I can't really see their face. That makes it hard, because then I don't feel like I'm getting any non-verbal communication from them really. In the past they've had me do hand signals. Just to tap my stomach if I need to step back for a second. We come up with little codes like that, but that hasn't always worked out in the past. If we come up with the code, and it seems clear, and then in the past I've had dentists not really be onboard with that, even if it's well communicated. I don't know maybe they just forget or this takes all of their attention being in my mouth. - Sophia'
Communicating ASD diagnosis	'Yes, the most recent one [dentist] does. I think it probably would've been helpful. Definitely would've been helpful in the past if I had the knowledge myself to be able to communicate that to dentists, or try to find one who had a specialty. But unfortunately, I didn't realize until the past year and a half. But it's been good information to be able to share since then. - Sophia'
	'I would rather they did know, mostly because they want to be able to get more experience on working with people like me so they'll know how to treat others that have autism, PDD-NOS and other symptoms such as that. - Quinn'
	'No, only because I don't want to be looked at as more different than any other patient that comes through. So, I don't really disclose anything that could be traumatic or could have myself looked in a different way than anybody else in there. - Rose'

Table 3.4 Oral self-care recommendations likes and dislikes

Emotional experience	Quote
Liking oral self-care	*'I like doing the floss, because it gets my teeth cleaned. That's the thing I liked the most and that tongue scraper. - Ethan'*
Neutral oral self-care	*'I never liked nor dislike it [daily oral hygiene], I know it's just something that I have to do. - David'*
Disliking oral self-care	*'I don't like mouthwash. I don't like using it. I don't like the taste of it, well, except cinnamon. Cinnamon that is the only exception. I do not like using mouthwash at all. - Kevin'*
	'I don't like a toothbrush in my mouth. I don't like thinking about my mouth. If I draw any attention to it then I'm feeling everything, and it's really unnerving. It didn't used to hurt, but now I have bad oral hygiene because now it does hurt to brush my teeth. But mostly it's just the pressure on my teeth. - Sophia'

Table 3.5 Sensory challenges during oral healthcare

Emotional experience	Quote
Auditory	*'It's both [the sound and the feel of all instruments and equipment]. Equally bad, I think it's hard to separate them but I think it's more the feeling. The sound of scraping is hard. I've tried to wear earplugs in the past, but that made the sound worse because it's in your head. So you can hear. Headphones would make it worse only because then I wouldn't know what is going to happen and what is happening because I wouldn't be able to hear it. - Sophia'*
	'If there's multiple people and they're having two different conversations at once that can be extremely disorienting. When there's just copious amounts of acoustic linguistic stimuli, I actually experience aphasia, with all that stimuli. If I'm trying to actually absorb it all at once, analyze every single detail, but that's impossible. - Karl'
Visual	*'One thing I don't like is how the light is always really bright. The light up above your head and you always have to close your eyes that is also when they're working. - Ethan'*
Tactile	*'Inside my mouth, the inside of my cheeks and my gums, it's like this electric pain. It just makes me want to scream. But I get desensitized to it as it goes along. It's not something that builds. Some of the things build, the tools that builds but just in general having this brushing inside of my mouth gets better as it goes. Outside it doesn't. Outside doesn't bother me too much but my lips and my gums on the inside of my mouth. - Sophia'*

discuss instances when they interacted with autistic patients in their practices, any adjustments that they made to their practice to accommodate the needs of their autistic patients, and any issues that arose during dental consultations. The data was analysed using thematic analysis, which produced four key themes:

1. the unique dental needs associated with being autistic,
2. effective adaptations to practice,

Table 3.6 Selection of themes from McMillion et al.'s (2022) study

Theme	Quote
Unique dental needs associated with being autistic	*'He basically didn't have "his cup" with "his juice", therefore he wouldn't take the pre-med, and we had to abandon the general anesthetic for that day... ... it really impressed on us the importance with severely autistic children of making sure that you're fully aware of any normal habits that they have, and making sure that you stick with their routine'*
Effective adaptations to practice	*'For a significant proportion of my children who have an autism diagnosis, it may take them a little bit longer, or significantly longer to attain, what I call dental life skills like, being able to enter the surgery, being able to sit in a chair, allow a dental exam, accept a toothbrush, accept fluoride varnish, accept air water suction and be able to understand why they're there and what's involved, put glasses on, put a bib on, and make that a normal part of their dental experience'*
The crucial role of the caregiver	*'Any parent or carer, they can vary, and you have someone very supportive, and will really sort of push you to get the best for their child or person that they're caring for but, others who aren't so helpful and might not persevere with the brushing, persevere with bringing them to the dental surgery so, lots of variation. Well, that's not the right word but other people that support and people who don't necessarily give as much support, and some are excellent'*
The importance of specialist knowledge	*'An awful lot of it, I've learnt by doing. You know, just by having encountered lots of patients in the autistic spectrum, you get the experience of "this worked before, we'll try this... we know this doesn't work". That sort of thing. And you start to recognize patterns in the patients, things you've encountered before'*

Source McMillion et al. (2022)

3. the crucial role of the caregiver, and
4. the importance of specialist knowledge (see Table 3.6).

Based on the insights from dental professionals that were collected and examined, McMillion and colleagues (2022, pp. 127–128) concluded that:

> To conclude, dental professionals experience a number of barriers when working with autistic patients, but they have developed many effective techniques to overcome them. The ability to implement these techniques is dependent on one's level of training, specialty and caregiver support. Above all else, recognizing that each autistic person is unique and has his/her own individualized needs is fundamental for the provision of effective care. Understanding the experiences of dental professionals can help improve access to dental care and address the unmet needs of autistic patients. Several recommendations from this study emerged based on the results. Dental professionals should include the autistic patient in decision making about their treatment plan whenever possible. Additionally, dental professionals should be willing to flexibly modify these plans as care continues. All dental professionals should have access to basic training about special care dentistry and autism at an undergraduate level, with specific hands-on training available for those who wish to avail themselves of it. Dentists should always be willing to work with autistic patients and their caregivers (who can provide valuable information and aid in treatment) and should be mindful of making secondary care referrals based solely on a diagnosis of autism.

3.2.3 What Experiences Have Parents Had with Their Autistic Child Receiving Dental Care?

In response to the question '*What experiences have parents had with their autistic child receiving dental care?*' searches of PubMed revealed seven studies that addressed this question (Erwin et al., 2022; Junnarkar et al., 2022; Kind et al., 2021; Logrieco et al., 2021; Parry et al., 2021; Stein Duker et al., 2019; Thomas et al., 2018).

The purpose of Erwin et al.'s (2022) systematic literature review was to examine studies about the factors that influence the oral health behaviours of autistics, as well as the literature about access to and delivery of dental care for autistic children and young people. From the 59 studies that were included, nine themes were identified, which were:

1. affordability and accessibility,
2. autism-related factors and cognitive or motor skill differences,
3. the dental environment,
4. managing autistic children and young people behaviour,
5. responding and adapting to the needs of the autistic children and young people and their parent/carer,
6. attitude of dental health professionals towards autistic children and young people and their parents/carers,
7. knowledge of how to care for and support autistic children and young people oral health,
8. empowerment of parents/carers and collaboration with dental health professionals, and
9. communication and building rapport.

Erwin et al.'s analysis of these studies yielded a wide selection of participant quotes about these nine themes (see Table 3.7).

Based on the collected insights from the participants in the reviewed studies Erwin and colleagues (2022) concluded that:

> The adoption of healthy OH [oral health] behaviours and access to dental care by autistic CYP [children and young people] is impacted by a range of factors including those intrinsically related to a diagnosis of autism, for example, communication and those often associated with autism, for example, sensory sensitivities. Access to better OH and dental care can be facilitated by responding to the individual needs of autistic CYP through accommodation, education and adaptation. This necessitates greater awareness and knowledge of autism amongst DHPs [dental health professionals] and the provision of appropriate services. More methodologically robust intervention studies are needed to identify effective ways to support autistic CYP in achieving good OH and access to dental care.

Due to sensory processing issues, demanding behaviours, and reported dentist reluctance to treat autistic children, it can be problematic for such children to receive preventative dental care. Thomas and colleagues (2018) conducted a study to learn about the dental experiences of autistic children from the perspective of their parents

Table 3.7 Quotes illustrating themes relating to factors influencing oral health behaviours, access to and provision of dental care

Themes	Relevant quotes from qualitative descriptive studies
Affordability and accessibility	Parent—'I was finally able to find a paediatric dental provider who was wonderful and [had] patience. However, our dental insurance would not cover the cost of that provider, as being a specialist; the insurance found it an unnecessary expense' (Hauschild et al., 2019)
	Parent—'Parent in a US study describing how, as soon as she thought her son had ASD, she '...changed my insurance from a HMO to a PPO because I knew if I stayed in the HMO it was going to be really hard to get a child-centred dentist, much less one with experience with special needs kids' (Stein Duker et al., 2017)
Autism-related factors and cognitive or motor skill difficulties	'I was totally unable to get into her mouth for the first several years of her life because she was so sensitive. She is also not communicative so it doesn't help to explain' (Lewis et al., 2015)
	'This was difficult. This was very difficult. We didn't use toothpaste for a long time. He had a very hard time with the taste. The taste was not appealing to him' (Abomriga, 2017)
	'Brushing teeth falls at the bottom of my priority list. There are so many stressors. We're all exhausted by the end of the day' (Lewis et al., 2015)
	'Due to his condition, we have to do a lot of things for him. So, the checklist is long and brushing teeth comes at the very end. Since both of us are working, by the time we completed the entire checklist, we wear ourselves out' (Rohani et al., 2018)
Managing children's behaviour	Parent—'My son is very sensory oriented... once he steps in that environment he feels uncomfortable... all the sensory devices will just make him so uncomfortable' (Stein Duker et al., 2017)
	Parent—'My son couldn't stand being touched. He was unable to follow multiple steps'
	'It was difficult because my child doesn't like to sit in the chair and doesn't like when the light is on'
	'She has so many sensory issues the light, the noise, and even the little things bug her...' (Hauschild et al., 2019)
	Parent—'...she'll usually be hyper on the way there, very hyper...and then as soon as we get there...she will just be back and forth to the toilet...often, her name will be called and she's in the toilet...she's just very stressed. Very, very anxious, very worried about what they're going to do' (Thomas et al., 2018)

(continued)

Table 3.7 (continued)

Themes	Relevant quotes from qualitative descriptive studies
	Dentist— 'Someone with ASD doesn't understand that you want to take care of his mouth and that it's a good thing that you scratch with a scaler, with a sound-producing, rotating machinery that develops vibrations and sounds, which perhaps by someone with ASD is experienced much stronger and more exciting than average people. This person sees it as a burden not as a possible benefit. So it scares them and they find it unpleasant, therefore they will repel' (Koojiman, 2016)
The attitude of DHPs towards autistic CYP and their parents/carers	Parent— 'There was a lot of eye rolling. People look at you like why can't you just discipline your kid out of it. They never explained anything to him...; the staff wasn't really trying, they weren't very warm or caring and they just gave up' (Hauschild et al., 2019)
	Parent— 'There have also been times when I felt like the hygienist would talk down to me because my son had a cavity, and really questioned how I enforce his brushing habits at home' (Hauschild et al., 2019)
	Parent— 'There's quite a snotty receptionist there'. I don't think she's at all child-friendly to be fair.... the slightest squeak that [my child] makes and she's on the phone and she's like, 'oh. Um. I'm sorry. I can hardly hear you, we've got some children in here, and they're being a bit naughty' (Thomas et al. 2018)
	Parent— '... A lot of positive reinforcement is helpful to my son, but I'm also going to throw in that it is helpful to me. It's important for me to see that the dentist is sensitive to my son and the way that it is and it just it doesn't faze her [the dentist] the same way it would someone else. Like he [my son] could be like completely melting [down] right there having like wanting to get out and you know it's embarrassing or like it gets very very tense and to see her [the dentist] just be understanding and not change and just keep at it and keep her positive reinforcement' (Stein Duker et al., 2019)
	Parent— 'I don't think she had any dealings with autism before that. I'm not sure she has now; you know, since. But I just think it was her open attitude and the fact that we said, 'look, is this.... you know, we want to do this, is this ok?' and she was like, 'yeah, absolutely'. So, it was her, completely her attitude, you know' (Thomas et al., 2018)
Knowledge of how to care for and support the child's oral health	Parent— 'It was a struggle to brush his teeth before. But after I met a dentist at the hospital, he taught me how to brush the back teeth. My child is now more cooperative during tooth brushing' (Rohani et al., 2018)

(continued)

Table 3.7 (continued)

Themes	Relevant quotes from qualitative descriptive studies
	Parent— 'We made an appointment for him to see that dentist. But she did not have any experience with special needs at all. So, she wasn't very good at handling him. He couldn't sit on the chair. He would run around the office. Just waiting at the waiting room…that is just not a very good experience for anyone in that way' (Abomriga, 2017)
The dental environment	Parent— 'Because the waiting room is a whole separate thing – it's almost like having an appointment in its own right, going and sitting in the waiting room – that's a thing, and then you go and do the dentist which is another big thing' (Stein Duker et al., 2019)
Responding and adapting to the needs of the autistic child and their parent/carer	Parent— 'I presented a whole thing at the school on toothbrushing at school so they would start to do that at school. I did because it was such a struggle at home, and I wanted someone else to be working on it, too, and for him to see his peers doing it' (Lewis et al., 2015)
	Parent— 'I am really pleased with the way our dentist works. The dentist started with a really, really slow routine to make him comfortable. The chair goes up and down. My son loves water and he loves to suck it up in the silly straw, and then they said, "let's look in your mouth and count your teeth". The first time they didn't get any cleaning done…it is still really hard to get his teeth cleaned' (Lewis et al., 2015)
	Parent— 'What helps my son is social stories, preparing him using a book I created called Going to the Dentist, with actual pictures of the dentist's office and the people he is going to see' (Lewis et al., 2015)
	Parent— 'With routine suddenly things will click…it is a big problem if she feels out of control and doesn't know what's coming next and negative experience is such a setback' (Parry & Shepherd, 2018)
The empowerment of parents/carers and collaboration with DHPs	Parent— 'I want them to ask: "what is the best way to proceed with your son?"'
	Parent— 'No one has really ever asked me, but I would be thrilled if someone wanted to know if there are special things we need to do differently because of his autism' (Lewis et al., 2015)
	Parent— 'Well, I suppose it's more of "we", as parents need to actually give them what works for our child or what our child – because with the autism and Asperger's, they're all so different – to have a blanket, "well this is what you need to do" I suppose is quite hard to do, but I mean, maybe it's more, the practice is saying "well let us know what we can do for you – what do you think is going to work for you?"' (Thomas et al., 2018)

(continued)

Table 3.7 (continued)

Themes	Relevant quotes from qualitative descriptive studies
Communication and building rapport	Parent— 'My son was unable to tell me if and when he had a toothache, or a blister, or anything else in his mouth' (Hauschild et al., 2019)
	Parent— 'They spoke to him in a very normal way. They didn't appear to be worried that he may not understand or not respond or do things as quickly as they wanted to. I actually found the experience was fantastic and the staff were very good in the way they managed someone like L. who has special needs' (Taghizadeh et al., 2019)
	Dentist— 'The bottleneck for me is that you don't get the usual feedback on direct contact. So you try to make contact and you try to get response so that you can continue to the next initiative, but in people with ASD it's often the case that you will not get the expected response and therefore you get lost in the moment. And not only you are lost as practitioner, but also the patient doesn't understand you and that's a big challenge' (Koojiman, 2016)
	Dentist— 'You often see when it's not clear what will happen, that someone who doesn't get all the pieces together will express himself with repetitive behaviour or defensive behaviour, because he is anxious since he doesn't understand what will come' (Koojiman, 2016)
	Dentist on establishing rapport—' … 'it's been very difficult when they've been four, five, six, or seven, and trying to manage them, but you know, they've kept coming back, they've been OK to come back and then they suddenly change and they become a bit more accepting of the treatment and they are still coming in and by the time they're ten, eleven, twelve, they love it!' (Parry & Shepherd, 2018)

Source Erwin et al. (2022, pp. 1275–1276)

in the UK and to discover how these parents think dental care services for their autistic children could be improved. For their study, semi-structured interviews with a total of 17 parents of autistic children or children pending an autistic diagnosis were conducted. The dental team's and the environment's adaptability, parents' confidence to speak out for their children's needs, service continuity, and clear referral paths to expert providers were the major themes that emerged. Additionally, experiences about the dentist's chair, waiting room difficulties, perceived medical authority, and the significance of ongoing treatment were also discovered. Thomas and colleagues concluded that in keeping with previous research about the value of family-centred care, a strong bond between parents and the entire dental team was necessary for autistic children to have dental exams and a positive dental experience.

Kind and colleagues (2021) examined if autistic children who lived in Holland routinely consulted a dentist and to gauge how satisfied their parents were with the dental treatment that their autistic children received. Parents of autistic children, who were aged 2–18 years, were asked to respond to a survey. The survey included questions about the degree of autism, the frequency of dental visits, the history of tooth discomfort, the kind of dental office, and the happiness of the parents. Of the 246 who completed the survey, 19 were rejected because of an incomplete or unconfirmed autistic diagnosis. All parents claimed that their autistic children went to the dentist at least once, and 5% had their last dental appointment more than a year ago. Additionally, 15% of autistic children did not obtain the necessary care when they suffered a toothache and 21% were dissatisfied with the dental care provided. There was no difference in the type of dental office attended between pleased and dissatisfied parents ($p > 0.05$). Dissatisfied parents reported higher discomfort in the previous year ($p = 0.013$) and had a more severe type of autism ($p = 0.016$). In summary, most parents of autistic children surveyed attended a dentist on a regular basis, and 21% of their parents were dissatisfied with the dental treatment that their autistic children received.

Drawing from the experiences and perspectives of their parents, Junnarkar and colleagues (2022) identified the obstacles to dental treatment for autistic children in Singapore. They conducted a focus group discussion and semi-structured interviews. All interviews were audio recorded, transcribed, and categorised into themes. In total, 23 parents raising autistic children 3 and 12 years of age participated. The following obstacles were identified:

1. Toothbrushing challenges and usage of inadequately fluoridated toothpaste among autistic children are caused by sensory, physical, and parental knowledge concerns,
2. Delayed dental visits due to parental concerns about managing the child, personal attitudes towards dentistry, lack of information on special needs dentist, and perceived high cost of dental treatment, and
3. Parental involvement and input for dental visits are essential to overcome challenges for dental visits (see Table 3.8).

Table 3.8 Themes identified by Junnarkar and colleagues (2022)

Main theme	Sub-theme	Quotes by parents of children aged 3–6 years	Quotes by parents of children aged 6–12 years
Toothbrushing challenges and usage of inadequately fluoridated toothpaste among autistic children are caused by sensory, physical, and parental knowledge concerns	Sensory issues affecting toothbrushing	'I try to let brush her teeth but she will bite her tooth brush. She will. so, all the tooth brushes all, [..], she will just bite in one, one area so, so I couldn't pull the tooth brush back'	'I think when bristles of the toothbrush is hard then he almost don't want to do it- he will just like scratch it and just throw away the toothbrush so I have to uh.. look for very soft bristles. The toothbrush like I mentioned earlier, we have quite a bit of problems when the bristles are hard. So actually I tried all the brands and I found none of them very good. Actually I'm very surprised that the bristles for the children's toothbrush are so hard. So in the end I went everywhere to buy. I went to like all the neighborhood shops, the Japanese shops and all that. So I found some that were very soft and they were made in Japan. But their problem is that they are not always available and not always the same shop will sell them so I'm always walking around buying toothbrushes'
	Problems with taste sensitivity, spitting out toothpaste, and rigidity about changing toothpaste	'We only use certain toothbrush and certain toothpaste. I cannot change the brand, I cannot change the flavour uh the toothpaste he is using. I think it's the Colgate one. I can't remember the flavour because I always buy the same thing so I never read but, must be that brand and that flavour. I cannot change, because I did change. There was a period of time I changed to stop that flavour. He refused to brush teeth during that period of time'	'Yes, it's the non-fluoride one and because of that we have, we have actually maintained that like until maybe like 5,6 years old; when actually he is supposed to change to a fluoride one. But we didn't. So, his teeth condition actually deteriorate during that time. Yes. Oh, because he has problem gargling. Gargling. So, so we figured that too much fluoride is bad for the body and then you know if he cannot throw it out then it will be all in the body and it will be bad, you know, for him. So, we stick on with the non-fluoride for very long time'

(continued)

Table 3.8 (continued)

Main theme	Sub-theme	Quotes by parents of children aged 3–6 years	Quotes by parents of children aged 6–12 years
Delayed dental visits due to parental concerns about managing the child, personal attitudes towards dentistry, lack of information on special needs dentist, and perceived high cost of dental treatment	Parental opinion of appropriate age for dental visits	'I don't think it's time yet, maybe because he's only 4! (laughs); maybe after 6. Maybe when he is a bit more aware of why he is doing it.[…] he listens but maybe he doesn't understand yet. So maybe in a few years' time he, he can understand'	'I think when they reach the age that you can explain the procedures to them. Like routine, no, step one you go in you do what- you can show them pictures. If they are too young they don't know what to expect inside, it will become like a foreign place with a stranger going into my mouth. Already they have like issues with eating you know, certain food and all that. Then suddenly some object goes in the mouth from a stranger, so isn't that worse, no?'
	Concerns about child's ability to cope with dental treatment	'Well uh one of his traits is that he is quite rigid and he doesn't like new experiences and he can't really stay still for long periods of times. So I don't think that he would be able to sit still in a dentist chair. So I have not uh. persisted on, I have not started looking'	'I don't know anything so I quite worried like what, what my child is going to do right. So, you know at home, don't really like open the mouth- how is he going to survive in the dentist's chair right for so long; need to open the mouth for so long. So, a lot of things go through in my mind. So that one is the most difficult part-the fear that like the special child is already sensitive, to how to make him like, compliant to the environment'
	Difficulty in finding a dentist who can treat children with ASD	'Through the support group we do have a few contacts available recommending this dentist or that dentist. It will be good if we have a list of like probably child-friendly or ASD friendly dentists around'	'I think I didn't see any like brochure about you know any dental care for special kids. I didn't see. So, if I had that information it'd be like better for me lah … and my friends also like other Mums ya so like I got one friends the kids are quite sensitive right so she, they don't know where to go for their dental service'

(continued)

Table 3.8 (continued)

Main theme	Sub-theme	Quotes by parents of children aged 3–6 years	Quotes by parents of children aged 6–12 years
	Concerns of cost of dental visits	*'I never bring him go to a dentist because I very scared that he don't open his mouth. Then because we go to private dentist, you need to pay a lot also even though he didn't do anything, right? [..] It's, it's no point to pay a lot and then he refuse to do anything. This is, this is my concern [..] is like no point go there then he is struggling, then you pay a big lump sum because he is struggling - I didn't even check the tooth'*	
PARENTAL QUOTES			
Parental involvement and input for dental visits are essential to overcome challenges for dental visits	Need for acclimation visits	*'I feel that the visit itself shouldn't start right away (laughs). They should let the child actually get used to the environment first because they will be very sensitive to a new environment so getting them to familiarise themselves in the room itself first before really starting on the whatever procedure or cleaning will be better at least they will not be having the kind of anxiety of where am I? Why this place – all the things are so unfamiliar. I don't even know if these things are going to harm me or not'*	
	Need for locally relevant information	*'If there is like a forum or a platform where there will be like all these books recommended that the parents can look up, some videos on Youtube or even YouTube is just like American, American references and all that. May be a local production, you know like a visit to the National dental centre. So that the kids know how it looks like because even like how I walk into the clinic, how the clinic looks like, who will be the people that I see, the receptionists and all that, waiting room what it looks like- having seen it first on the video I can prepare myself- my anxiety level goes down [...]-having someone like maybe my son for example, an ASD kid who is okay with doing all this dental treatments and is shown. Ya. That might help. In Chinese, in Malay, or different languages'*	

(continued)

Table 3.8 (continued)

Main theme	Sub-theme	Quotes by parents of children aged 3–6 years	Quotes by parents of children aged 6–12 years
	Strategies for preparing for dental visits	'I took him to the library and I showed him books about people going to the dentist and the kind of instruments they use, like you know like that mirror – it's round with that sharp thing that scrapes– I don't know the names of those things but you know I just show it to him and I kind of like enacted it out, you know'	
	Modifications to the dental environment		'He doesn't exactly tell me what it is but I suspect that that would be too many visuals on the wall or lighting that could cause him to feel more anxious because he has to filter all these things and he doesn't know what's coming up'
	Parental input is essential	'We needed to count, because the doctor didn't count for him and so he got stressed. Ya so then – so one help was we were all in the room and so we told the doctor you cannot just ask him to open the mouth and put the tool in because he cannot- he doesn't know when it's going to end and so that stresses him. So, we told him we must take it out- we have to count to 20'	
	Desirable qualities of dental team		'I also think that the dentist cannot keep changing, he must always be a familiar figure because if let's say this year I see this lady next year another dentist comes in but it's a totally different person – to them they need familiarity'

Notes All quotes appear as originally found, without edits [sic]. Quotes are followed by parent identification codes. In all quotes, square brackets containing an ellipsis [..] indicate short portions of omitted speech
Source Junnarkar et al. (2022)

To identify interventions that will promote positive experiences with dental attendance, Parry and colleagues (2021) sought to examine parental perceptions of challenges related to dental attendance and oral care for autistic children and young adults. They also aimed to discover reported challenges and potential adaptations. Qualitative data was acquired from two focus groups with parents of autistic elementary and secondary school students. Parents' attitudes of dental attendance and oral care were elicited. The focus groups were audio recorded and verbatim transcribed. The transcripts were evaluated and preliminary codes were developed. Thematic analysis yielded the development of subthemes and themes. Parental perspectives included the requirement for education and training, understanding sensory issues, and acknowledgement of the uniqueness of autistic traits. These perceptions supported the findings from other studies. Participants in the focus groups emphasised the usefulness of emphasising an autistic perspective and the significance of spreading optimistic oral health messaging. The difficulty of changing self-imposed, ritualistic food regimens and striving to instil healthy oral preventative behaviours among autistic children.

Some autistics have severe dental issues, yet there are only a few studies about effective methods to enhance their dental health. Stein Duker and colleagues (2019) investigated parental and dental experiences about beneficial measures used during dental treatment for autistic children. Two focus groups were held with parents of autistic children and two focus groups were held with dentists who treat autistic children. The focus group discussions were audio recorded, transcribed, and then thematically analysed to identify the themes in the transcripts. An examination of the transcripts from the focus group of parents yielded three themes, which were (1) what makes a good dentist; (2) flexibility and techniques-strategies used by the dentist; and (3) preparation-strategies for parents and caregivers of autistic children. Four themes were identified after an examination of the transcripts of the focus group of dentists, which were (1) parents know best; (2) practice; (3) flexibility; and (4) a network of colleagues. The importance of preparation, necessity of flexibility and creativity, and value of collaboration were themes that were identified between both the focus groups of parents and dentists. Based on these results, Stein Duker and colleagues (2019, p. 12) concluded that:

> Parents and dental professionals repeatedly discussed the importance of preparation both for the home and dental environments. In the home, preparation centered on practicing activities to take place during dental visits by watching videos, reading books, and using visual schedules or step-by-step lists of oral care activities. In the dental office, preparation focused on multiple desensitization appointments where the child could visit the office prior to the cleaning. The utilization of these types of preparation activities have previously been reported, with 71% of dentist members of the Special Care Dentistry Association who treated patients with ASD offering familiarization visits.

Providing oral healthcare to autistic children can pose significant challenges for the child, their family, and the dentist. The purpose of Logrieco et al.'s (2021) study was to investigate and understand the difficulties experienced by these three parties during oral care treatment. Their study involved the completion of two separate multiple-choice questionnaires by a cohort of 275 parents of non-autistic children,

57 parents of autistic children aged 3–15 years, and 61 dentists. The results indicated that both parents and dentists found it challenging to provide dental treatment to autistic children, primarily due to demographic factors of the caregivers, issues encountered before and during dental exams, and a shortage of experts in autism-specific treatment.

3.2.4 What Barriers Prevent Autistics from Receiving Dental Care?

In response to the question '*What barriers prevent autistics from receiving dental care?*' searches of PubMed revealed seven studies that addressed this question (AlHumaid, 2022; Alshatrat et al., 2020; Alshihri et al., 2021; Alvares et al., 2022; Bernath & Kanji, 2021; Du et al., 2019; Mansoor et al., 2018).

Alshatrat and colleagues (2020) assessed the usage of dental services in Jordan among autistics and identified obstacles to dental treatment that they encountered compared to non-autistics. A case-control study was conducted with 296 parents/caregivers who were raising autistic or non-autistic children, who completed a self-designed questionnaire. Most respondents in both groups had consulted with a dentist during the year preceding the completion of the questionnaire. Addressing their child's toothache was the most common reason for visiting a dental service (43%). In contrast, the least common cause (11.6%) was a routine check-up. Autistic children were substantially more likely than non-autistic children to experience a lack of specialised dental personnel (28.6%), a lack of understanding of how to manage people with impairments (26.6%), and insufficient facilities (34%) (see Table 3.9). They concluded that identifying and understanding the limitations to dental care access for autistics may enhance their overall oral health.

Alshihri et al.'s (2021) study had two objectives: first, to look at the challenges that parents had in getting their autistic children to dental care; second, to assess the factors that affect their ability to get these services. For their study, 142 mothers of autistic children completed a questionnaire. Finding dental treatment was challenging, according to 68.3% of respondents. The three biggest obstacles were cost (75.4%), finding a dentist who could treat their autistic child (74.6%), and their autistic child's conduct (45.1%). Medical insurance and prior negative experiences both significantly impacted how difficult it was to get dental care ($p = 0.05$).

Autistic children are more inclined to experience poor oral health and difficulty receiving oral medical services in comparison with non-autistic children. However, it is yet uncertain which autistic children are more inclined to experience challenges with dental care. Alvares and colleagues (2022) examined parental reports of autistic children's dental care needs as well as their relationships with different autistic phenotypes. In total, 140 parents raising autistic children who had taken part in the Australian Autism Biobank, a major national biobank project, completed a survey about their autistic child's oral health, service utilisation, and obstacles to

Table 3.9 Barriers to dental care among participants with ASD and control groups

Barrier	ASD, N (%)	Control, N (%)	p value
Could not afford the cost	64 (43.5)	57 (38.3)	0.058
Dental office is too far away	39 (26.5)	19 (12.8)	0.003*
Dental office is not open at convenient times	34 (23.1)	40 (26.8)	0.460
Dental office has no or difficult access for wheelchair	61 (41.5)	10 (6.7)	0.001*
Dental office has inaccessible parking areas	52 (35.4)	9 (6.0)	0.001*
Dental office has a small space	42 (28.6)	7 (4.8)	0.001*
Dental office has inadequate facilities to provide dental care	50 (34)	5 (3.4)	0.001*
Dentist's lack of knowledge of how to treat people with disability	42 (26.6)	9 (6.1)	0.001*
Dental office has a general dentist, not a specialist	42 (28.6)	14 (9.4)	0.001*
Long waiting time	72 (49)	62 (41.6)	0.203
Fear of dental work	99 (67.3)	77 (51.7)	0.006*
No insurance coverage/dental coverage	57 (39)	52 (34.9)	0.461
Embarrassment or any psychological barriers	64 (43.5)	14 (9.4)	0.001*

Notes * Significant result, $p < 0.05$
Source Alshatrat et al. (2020, p. 5)

care. One-third of respondents disclosed that their child's dental health was poorer than that of other children their age, with 26% reporting untreated dental issues. Additionally, a third of autistic children were found to have received general anesthesia for dental treatments at least once. However, autistic children with intellectual impairments and functional issues were more inclined to have general anesthesia. Finally, parents of autistic children with severe functional limits and sensory issues reported more barriers to receiving dental treatment. The findings have significant ramifications for paediatric dentists who treat autistic children who also have intellectual, functional, and sensory difficulties. Their findings may guide the creation of more individualised assistance for people with autism.

Bernath and Kanji (2021) published a narrative review that highlighted the unique demands that autistics have when seeking dental treatment and to highlight potential ways to remove obstacles to such care. They reviewed 21 articles that had a variety of research types and methodology. Behavioural problems, limited social and communication skills, parental dependency, clinical settings, and the ability of oral health professionals to serve patients with specific care requirements were major themes that surfaced as care obstacles. According to the reviewed research, autistics encounter severe obstacles when trying to receive dental treatment and maintain good oral health, which adds to the burden of illness. To reduce the obstacles to treatment that these communities encounter, oral health practitioners should endeavour to increase awareness among other healthcare providers and enhance their understanding of special care populations like those in the autistic community.

To research the difficulties experienced by autistic children and their families in Dubai, Mansoor and colleagues (2018) conducted a case–control comparison study involving 84 autistic children and 53 non-autistic children, including siblings of the autistic children. Parents or guardians complete a survey form, which was used to collect the data. Compared to parents raising non-autistic children, more parents of autistic children reported that their children had difficulty with practically every aspect of oral hygiene. For example, 15.4% of parents raising non-autistic children and 83.3% of parents raising autistic children reported that their children required help with brushing their teeth. Additionally, the parents of autistic children reported that their children were more recalcitrant during dental appointments and substantially more of these parents gave their child's visit a bad review than did the parents of non-autistic children. According to their results, autistic children in Dubai have greater difficulties and obstacles when it comes to dental hygiene than non-autistic children.

Du and colleagues (2019) assessed the oral health behaviours and obstacles to dental care in preschool autistics and non-autistic children as well as their parents' dental knowledge and attitudes. Those raising autistic children reported greater rates for several environmental barriers to dental treatment compared to parents raising non-autistic children. Examples of environmental barriers were:

- Difficulty finding a dentist willing to treat my child because of his/her medical condition (48.9% ASD parental group vs. 8.1% non-ASD parental group).
- Difficulty travelling to the dental office (3.3% ASD parental group vs. 3.2% non-ASD parental group).
- Difficulty finding a dentist for my child near my home (17.5% ASD parental group vs. 4% non-ASD parental group).
- Difficulty finding a dentist that will accept my child's dental insurance (11.5% ASD parental group vs. 5.6% non-ASD parental group).
- Dental staff feeling anxious about giving my child dental treatment (16.4% ASD parental group vs. 6.5% non-ASD parental group).

Parents of autistic children also reported greater rates for several non-environmental barriers to receiving dental care for their autistic children when compared to parents raising non-autistic children. Examples of these non-environmental barriers were:

- My child is afraid of the dentist (40.7% ASD parental group vs. 38.7% non-ASD parental group).
- My child does not like any procedure done in their mouth (63.7% ASD parental group vs. 39.5% non-ASD parental group).
- My child cannot behave cooperatively at the dentist (59.9% ASD parental group vs. 25% non-ASD parental group).

- My child's medical conditions make dental treatment very complicated (11.5% ASD parental group vs. 0.8% non-ASD parental group).
- My child has other more urgent healthcare needs (17% ASD parental group vs.3. 5% non-ASD parental group).

3.3 Limitations of the Current Research

3.3.1 Experiences Autistics Have Had in Dental Clinics

An examination of the citations retrieved from the four separate searched of PubMed revealed two studies that could be used to answer the question '*What experiences have autistics had in dental clinics?*' (McMillion et al., 2021; Mirsky et al., 2021). Several limitations in these two studies were explained by their authors. McMillion and colleagues (2021) acknowledged that they distributed their survey throughout the entire UK. However, despite its distribution, most responses that they received came from people who lived in the South and Central areas of England. Thus, respondents from Scotland, Wales, and Northern Ireland were not adequately represented. Another limitation recognised by McMillion and colleagues was that only responses from people who could access the survey online participated. Mirsky and colleagues (2021) disclosed that their results were based on a small sample of young autistic adults (i.e., $n = 15$). Another limitation of their study was that autistics who did not have oral healthcare treatment within the past two years were not represented.

Three modifications to the design of studies in the future can be made to ensure that we develop a more accurate understanding about the experiences that autistics have in dental clinics. First, researchers in the future should distribute their surveys to a broader geographical section of the community instead of localising its distribution to specific areas. Disseminating the survey within a broader geographical area will ensure that the results can be better generalised. Second, respondents should be given the opportunity to complete the study's survey in paper form instead of only being given the option to complete it electronically. Similarly, respondents should be given other opportunities to express their views, such as being interviewed. Third, to improve the generalisability of the results collected studies in the future should have larger sample sizes. Such studies will address the limitation embedded within the study published by Mirsky and colleagues.

3.3.2 Experiences Dentists Have Had with Treating Autistics

An analysis of the citations generated from the four separate searches of PubMed revealed two studies that were deemed to answer the question '*What experiences have dentists had with treating autistics?*' (Eades et al., 2019; McMillion et al., 2022). Eades and colleagues (2019) collected data at one specific point in time. Hence, longitudinal data was not collected and examined. Despite their study's contributions, McMillion and colleagues (2022) explained that their results were only based on a relatively small sample of 16 participants who primarily worked with paediatric patients. Such a small sample hampered the ability to apply the results to a broader cohort of dentists. Another limitation of McMillion and colleagues' study was that half of the dentists interviewed had a personal interest and/or connection to autism which suggests a response bias towards those with a better understanding of autistic patients than the broader population of dentists. In the future studies should contain larger sample sizes so that the results collected can be better generalised. Studies should also ensure that their sample does not contain an overrepresentation of dentists who are familiar with autism since this overrepresentation would distort our judgement about the level of knowledge of autism among those in the dental profession.

3.3.3 Experiences Parents Have Had with Their Autistic Child Receiving Dental Care

In response to the question '*What experiences have parents had with their autistic child receiving dental care?*' seven studies were identified from the four separate PubMed searches (Erwin et al., 2022; Junnarkar et al., 2022; Kind et al., 2021; Logrieco et al., 2021; Parry et al., 2021; Stein Duker et al., 2019; Thomas et al., 2018). Within these seven studies, the authors explained the limitations in their research. For their mixed-methods systematic review, Erwin and colleagues (2022) only examined studies that were conducted in countries that had a high human development index. Studies conducted in countries with low human development index scores were not included in their study. The omission of such studies has the potential to skew the results examined. Logrieco and colleagues (2021), Kind and colleagues (2021), and Thomas and colleagues (2018) claimed that their studies had small sample sizes. Kind and colleagues sampled 227 respondents, Thomas and colleagues sampled 17 respondents, and Logrieco and colleagues sampled 275 parents of non-autistic children, 57 parents of autistic children aged 3–15 years, and 61 dentists. Small sample sizes have the potential to reduce the generalisability of the results produced. Junnarkar and colleagues and Thomas and colleagues both acknowledged that most participants in their study were mothers raising autistic children. The lack of fathers and other family members (e.g., grandparents) has resulted in the results being simplified and unable to be generalised to parents other than mothers raising autistic children. Stein Ducker and colleagues disclosed that those in the parent group of their study were not required to verify that their child was autistic. Another limitation in their study was that all parents had male children and that the experiences of parents taking their autistic daughters to a dentist were not explored.

To improve our understanding about the experiences that parents have when their autistic child is receiving dental care studies in the future should adopt the following four design modifications. First, respondents other than mothers of autistic children should be recruited so that this will correct the limitations identified by Junnarkar and colleagues and Thomas and colleagues. Second, sample sizes should be enlarged so that the results can be better generalised. Increasing the study's sample size would address the limitations in the studies published by Kind and colleagues and Thomas and colleagues. Third, before a parent participates in a study, they should be obligated to provide sufficient documentation that their child is autistic. This paperwork will correct the limitation revealed by Stein Ducker and colleagues. Fourth, parents who raise autistic daughters should be recruited and asked to describe the experiences that their daughters have had in dental clinics. Their insights will correct the deficiency in the study published by Stein Ducker and colleagues.

3.3.4 Barriers that Prevent Autistics from Receiving Dental Care

An examination of the citations retrieved from the four separate searched of PubMed revealed seven studies that could be used to answer the question 'What barriers prevent autistics from receiving dental care?' (AlHumaid, 2022; Alshatrat et al., 2020; Alshihri et al., 2021; Alvares et al., 2022; Bernath & Kanji, 2021; Du et al., 2019; Mansoor et al., 2018).

Several limitations in these studies were explained by their authors. For their literature review, AlHumaid (2022) did not include the insights contained within grey data and government reports. Alshatrat and colleagues (2020) only recruited autistics who attended special care centres. Additionally, information was only collected from self-reported questionnaires, which meant that the insights collected could not be validated using other people's views. Alshihri and colleagues (2021) claimed that their sample size was small and so the results collected could not be generalised to the entire autistic population. Alvares and colleagues (2022) relied on parental recollections, and consequently, they did not confirm these insights using dental examinations or hospital records. Alvares and colleagues also admitted that they mainly collected insights from people in middle to high income families who generally had less socioeconomic disadvantage relative to the Australian population. Mansoor and colleagues (2018) admitted that they only obtained data from parents of autistic children whose children went to a special needs school. Thus, the generalisability of their results and the truthfulness of the results collected could not be accomplished.

To overcome these design limitations, studies in the future about the barriers that prevent autistics from receiving dental care should incorporate three modifications. First, the size of the sample should increase so that the results collected can be better generalised. Second, the insights provided by the study's participants should be confirmed by comparing them with other stakeholders, such as dentists, and by other sources of information, such as dental reports. Third, researchers should ensure that they collect data from participants across the entire socioeconomic continuum. By adopting these strategies, the quality of research and our understanding about the barriers that prevent autistics from receiving dental care will improve.

3.4   Strategies to Assist Autistics in Dental Settings

3.4.1   Explaining the Dental Procedure Before It Commences

> Probably letting me know the steps as a process going between each step. Now I'm going to do this, and then complete that step and then move on to the next one and let me know what's going on as we go through the process. – Rose. (Mirsky et al., 2021, p. 47)

In the above quote Rose, an autistic participant in Mirsky et al.'s (2021) study, explained that to subdue her anxiety she expressed a preference for the dentist to explain all dental procedures before they commenced. To alleviate the uncertainty that autistics have about the upcoming dental procedure dentists should explain each part of the procedure and systematically check that the autistic patient understands the step. If plausible, the dentist could also reassure the autistic patient by talking about each step as they conduct it during the dental procedure.

3.4.2   Giving Autistic Patients the Opportunity to Become Familiar with Dental Instruments

> If the kids can lay hands on the instruments that the dentists have, that they can touch maybe not the metallic ones but the plastic you know like those kiddie ones that you buy from the supermarket that you pretend that you are a dentist, if they can have those and let the parents may be let them touch those things and play them around with it may be it will be more comfortable for them when they see the dentist holding them because they have already touched those things in their normal play. (Junnarkar et al., 2022)

Giving autistic patients the opportunity to physically examine medical and dental instruments can help reduce the anxiety and stress that they experience whilst undergoing dental examinations. Although this approach can help some autistics, it does pose a hygienic challenge for dentists. To ensure that their instruments remain sterile dentists can give their autistic patients instruments that they will not be using. Alternatively, as a participant in Junnarkar et al.'s (2022) study suggests, dentists can give the autistic patient fake dental equipment so that they have a familiarity with the real dental equipment during the dental procedure.

3.4.3 Giving Autistic Patients Visual Instructions About Dental Procedures

> If you are looking after children with autism, it's good that you have visuals for them like sit down open your mouth or things like that where they can see the picture and then they will follow the instruction. Yes, because sometimes the instruction comes a lot and they are overwhelmed and then of course the finish you know, (laughs)- yes. (Junnarkar et al., 2022)

Some autistic patients obtain information visually instead of from verbal instructions. To assist those autistics who are visual learners it would be advantageous for dentists to give them visual instructions. For example, a dentist could show an autistic patient a brief video about what they will do to clean their teeth. Such an instructional video would contain animations of a patient's mouth and an explanation and visual illustration of the dental instruments that will be used.

3.4.4 Giving Autistic Patients and/or Their Parents a Clinic Satisfaction Survey

To improve the experiences that autistic patients have in dental clinics, dentists should continuously re-evaluate their techniques and procedures. Giving autistic patients and their families a clinical satisfaction survey can help dentists and practice managers identify areas for improvement with the delivery of dental services for autistic patients. For their study, Weir and colleagues (2022) distributed a survey to autistic respondents about their experiences receiving medical assistance. Their survey has been adjusted so that it can be used by dentists and medical doctors to obtain feedback from autistic patients (see Appendix 2.2).

3.4.5 Removing Sensory Sensitivities from the Dental Environment

As explained in the previous chapter, some autistics have claimed that within clinical environments their sensory sensitivities can hamper their ability to obtain satisfactory medical treatment (Brice et al., 2021; Fallea et al., 2022; Weir et al., 2022). Mirsky and colleagues (2021) explained that similar sensory sensitivities have prevented some autistics from receiving dental treatment.

> The smell can be a little bit unusual. So, I would have scents like... more pleasant scents in the office, like a sweet lavender smell; and it would also help to calm someone down, especially if they're a little less comfortable around being in the dentist's office. – Quinn. (Mirsky et al., 2021, p. 47)

To ensure that autistic patients can receive adequate dental treatment and care their sensory sensitivities need to be dulled. To achieve this objective dentists and practice managers can ask autistic patients to complete a clinical satisfaction survey. The results of this survey can be used to modify dental procedures and the clinical environment to better accommodate the sensory needs of autistic patients (Weir et al., 2022) (see Appendix 2.2).

3.4.6   Giving Autistic Patients a Form for Them to Explain Their Dental Needs

Autistic patients can complete a form that can help dentists understand their dental needs and challenges. As explained in the previous chapter, the *National Autistic Society* has created a *My Health Passport*, a form that autistics can complete to inform medical doctors about their healthcare needs. Dentists can use a modified version of this form to help them understand the dental needs and challenges of their autistic patients (see Appendix 2.3).

3.4.7   Educating Dental Students About Autism

As expressed in the previous chapter, medical students have reported that medical school did not prepare them for assisting autistic patients (Austriaco et al., 2019; Clarke & Fung, 2022; Low & Zailan, 2016). A similar claim was made by several dentists in Mac Giolla Phadraig et al.'s (2022) study. To ensure that dental students in the future are adequately prepared to assist autistic patients it is vital that dental schools give dental students opportunities to learn about autism and strategies that they can use to effectively interact with autistic patients. Such learning opportunities can be created by asking autistic adults to describe to a class of dental students what it is like to be autistic and undergo dental procedures. Similarly, lecturers who teach students, such as psychology students, about the autism spectrum could be invited to present a lecture to dental students about the autism spectrum and some strategies to help autistics receive the best possible dental care.

3.4.8   Using Information and Communication Technologies

Autistic children tend to exhibit poorer oral health than their non-autistic peers and often have limited access to high-quality healthcare services. Narzisi et al.'s (2020) study aimed to describe an experience of dental care supported by Information and Communication Technologies for autistic children in a public health service. The

MyDentist project was implemented, which integrated traditional dental care techniques with new practices for desensitisation and fear control delivered through a customised Information and Communication Technology-based intervention. Their study included 59 autistic children, with an average age of 9.9 years, who participated in the project. Parents filled out two questionnaires to evaluate the acceptability of the MyDentist experience for their children. The results showed significant improvements in oral hygiene and cooperation during dental treatments from before the initiation of the MyDentist project to six months later. Parents positively assessed the use of Information and Communication Technology support, indicating that public health dental care and prevention can be successfully implemented without costly pharmacological interventions, taking better care of children's health.

3.5   Conclusion

This chapter started with a summary of the collected literature that answered the research questions about autistics in dental settings. This was followed by a selection that outlined the limitations in the reviewed literature. The final section explained some of the strategies that can help autistics participate in dental examinations and procedures. The section's purpose was to answer the research question '*What strategies can be used to help autistics attend dental and medical clinics?*'.

References

Abomriga, A. (2017). *Between struggle and hope: Understanding the oral care experiences of children living with Autism Spectrum Disorder (ASD): A parent's perspective.* Thesis. McGill University.

AlHumaid, J. (2022). Dental experiences related to oral care of children with autism spectrum disorders in Saudi Arabia: A literature review. *The Saudi Dental Journal, 34*(1), 1–10. https://doi.org/10.1016/j.sdentj.2021.09.023

Alshatrat, S. M., Al-Bakri, I. A., & Al-Omari, W. M. (2020). dental service utilization and barriers to dental care for individuals with autism spectrum disorder in jordan: A case-control study. *International Journal of Dentistry, 2020*, 3035463. https://doi.org/10.1155/2020/3035463

Alshihri, A. A., Al-Askar, M. H., & Aldossary, M. S. (2021). Barriers to professional dental care among children with autism spectrum disorder. *Journal of Autism and Developmental Disorders, 51*(8), 2988–2994. https://doi.org/10.1007/s10803-020-04759-y

Alvares, G. A., Mekertichian, K., Rose, F., Vidler, S., & Whitehouse, A. J. O. (2022). Dental care experiences and clinical phenotypes in children on the autism spectrum. *Special Care in Dentistry: Official Publication of the American Association of Hospital Dentists, the Academy of Dentistry for the Handicapped, and the American Society for Geriatric Dentistry, 43*(1), 17–28. https://doi.org/10.1111/scd.12746

Austriaco, K., Aban, I., Willig, J., & Kong, M. (2019). Contemporary trainee knowledge of autism: How prepared are our future providers? *Frontiers in Pediatrics, 7*, 165. https://doi.org/10.3389/fped.2019.00165

Bernath, B., & Kanji, Z. (2021). Exploring barriers to oral health care experienced by individuals living with autism spectrum disorder. *Canadian Journal of Dental Hygiene, 55*(3), 160–166.

Brice, S., Rodgers, J., Ingham, B., Mason, D., Wilson, C., Freeston, M., Le Couteur, A., & Parr, J. R. (2021). The importance and availability of adjustments to improve access for autistic adults who need mental and physical healthcare: Findings from UK surveys. *BMJ Open, 11*(3), e043336. https://doi.org/10.1136/bmjopen-2020-043336

Clarke, L., & Fung, L. K. (2022). The impact of autism-related training programs on physician knowledge, self-efficacy, and practice behavior: A systematic review. *Autism: The International Journal of Research and Practice, 26*(7), 1626–1640. https://doi.org/10.1177/136236132211 02016

Du, R. Y., Yiu, C. K. Y., & King, N. M. (2019). Oral health behaviours of preschool children with autism spectrum disorders and their barriers to dental care. *Journal of Autism and Developmental Disorders, 49*(2), 453–459. https://doi.org/10.1007/s10803-018-3708-5

Eades, D., Leung, P., Cronin, A., Monteiro, J., Johnson, A., & Remington, A. (2019). UK dental professionals' knowledge, experience and confidence when treating patients on the autism spectrum. *British Dental Journal, 227*(6), 504–510. https://doi.org/10.1038/s41415-019-0786-5

Erwin, J., Paisi, M., Neill, S., Burns, L., Vassallo, I., Nelder, A., Facenfield, J., Devalia, U., Vassallo, T., & Witton, R. (2022). Factors influencing oral health behaviours, access and delivery of dental care for autistic children and adolescents: A mixed-methods systematic review. *Health Expectations: An International Journal of Public Participation in Health Care and Health Policy, 25*(4), 1269–1318. https://doi.org/10.1111/hex.13544

Fallea, A., Zuccarello, R., Roccella, M., Quatrosi, G., Donadio, S., Vetri, L., & Calì, F. (2022). Sensory-adapted dental environment for the treatment of patients with autism spectrum disorder. *Children (Basel, Switzerland), 9*(3), 393. https://doi.org/10.3390/children9030393

Hauschild, J. L., Rainchuso, L., Boyd, L. D., & Smallidge, D. (2019). The experiences of caregivers when seeking and/or receiving oral health care for their child with autism. *Journal of Disability and Oral Health, 20*(2), 67–72.

Junnarkar, V. S., Tong, H. J., Hanna, K. M. B., Aishworiya, R., & Duggal, M. (2022). Qualitative study on barriers and coping strategies for dental care in autistic children: Parents' perspective. *International Journal of Paediatric Dentistry, 33*(3), 203–215. https://doi.org/10.1111/ipd. 13035

Kind, L. S., Aartman, I. H. A., van Gemert-Schriks, M. C. M., & Bonifacio, C. C. (2021). Parents' satisfaction on dental care of Dutch children with Autism Spectrum Disorder. *European Archives of Paediatric Dentistry: Official Journal of the European Academy of Paediatric Dentistry, 22*(3), 491–496. https://doi.org/10.1007/s40368-020-00586-y

Koojiman, R. (2016). *Barriers in oral hygiene in children with an autism spectrum disorder of various cultural backgrounds in the Netherlands*. Thesis. Vrije Universiteit Amsterdam.

Lewis, C., Vigo, L., Novak, L., & Klein, E. J. (2015). Listening to parents: A qualitative look at the dental and oral care experiences of children with autism spectrum disorder. *Pediatric Dentistry, 37*(7), E98–E104.

Logrieco, M. G. M., Ciuffreda, G. N., Sinjari, B., Spinelli, M., Rossi, R., D'Addazio, G., Lionetti, F., Caputi, S., & Fasolo, M. (2021). What happens at a dental surgery when the patient is a child with autism spectrum disorder? An Italian study. *Journal of Autism and Developmental Disorders, 51*(6), 1939–1952. https://doi.org/10.1007/s10803-020-04684-0

Low, H. M., & Zailan, F. (2016). Medical students' perceptions, awareness, societal attitudes and knowledge of autism spectrum disorder: An exploratory study in Malaysia. *International Journal of Developmental Disabilities, 64*(2), 86–95. https://doi.org/10.1080/20473869.2016.1264663

Mac Giolla Phadraig, C., Kahatab, A., & Daly, B. (2022). Promoting openness to autism amongst dental care professional students. *European Journal of Dental Education: Official Journal of the Association for Dental Education in Europe, 27*(2), 396–401. https://doi.org/10.1111/eje. 12821

Mansoor, D., Al Halabi, M., Khamis, A. H., & Kowash, M. (2018). Oral health challenges facing Dubai children with Autism Spectrum Disorder at home and in accessing oral health care.

European Journal of Paediatric Dentistry, 19(2), 127–133. https://doi.org/10.23804/ejpd.2018. 19.02.06

McMillion, A., Van Herwegen, J., Johnson, A., Monteiro, J., Cronin, A. J., & Remington, A. (2021). Dental experiences of a group of autistic adults based in the United Kingdom. *Special Care in Dentistry: Official Publication of the American Association of Hospital Dentists, the Academy of Dentistry for the Handicapped, and the American Society for Geriatric Dentistry, 41*(4), 474–488. https://doi.org/10.1111/scd.12583

McMillion, A., Tobiansky, B., Wang, K., Cronin, A. J., Johnson, A., Monteiro, J., & Remington, A. (2022). UK-based specialist dental professionals' experiences of working with autistic patients. *Special Care in Dentistry: Official Publication of the American Association of Hospital Dentists, the Academy of Dentistry for the Handicapped, and the American Society for Geriatric Dentistry, 42*(2), 120–136. https://doi.org/10.1111/scd.12653

Mirsky, L. B., Rogo, E. J., & Gurenlian, J. R. (2021). Oral care experiences of young adults with autism spectrum disorder. *Journal of Dental Hygiene, 95*(4), 41–50.

Mohamed-Rohani, M., Baharozaman, N. F., Khalid, N. S., & Ab-Murat, N. (2018). Autism spectrum disorder: Patients' oral health behaviors and barriers in oral care from parents' perspectives. *Annals of Dentistry, 25*(2), 43–52. https://doi.org/10.22452/adum.vol25no2.5

Narzisi, A., Bondioli, M., Pardossi, F., Billeci, L., Buzzi, M. C., Buzzi, M., Pinzino, M., Senette, C., Semucci, V., Tonacci, A., Uscidda, F., Vagelli, B., Giuca, M. R., & Pelagatti, S. (2020). "Mom let's go to the dentist!" Preliminary feasibility of a tailored dental intervention for children with autism spectrum disorder in the Italian public health service. *Brain Sciences, 10*(7), 444. https://doi.org/10.3390/brainsci10070444

Parry, J., & Shepherd, J. (2018). Understanding oral health challenges for children and young people with autistic spectrum conditions: Views of families and the dental team. *Journal of Disability and Oral Health, 19*(4), 170–174.

Parry, J. A., Newton, T., Linehan, C., & Ryan, C. (2021). Dental visits for autistic children: A qualitative focus group study of parental perceptions. *JDR Clinical and Translational Research*, 23800844211049404. Advance online publication. https://doi.org/10.1177/238008 44211049404

Rohani, M. M., Baharozaman, N. F., Khalid, N. S., & Ab-Murat, N. (2018). Autism spectrum disorder: Patients' oral health behaviors and barriers in oral care from parents' perspectives. *Annals of Dentistry*, 43–52.

Stein Duker, L. I. S., Henwood, B. F., Bluthenthal, R. N., Juhlin, E., Polido, J. C., & Cermak, S. A. (2017). Parents' perceptions of dental care challenges in male children with autism spectrum disorder: An initial qualitative exploration. *Research in Autism Spectrum Disorders, 39*, 63–72. https://doi.org/10.1016/j.rasd.2017.03.002

Stein Duker, L. I., Floríndez, L. I., Como, D. H., Tran, C. F., Henwood, B. F., Polido, J. C., & Cermak, S. A. (2019). Strategies for success: A qualitative study of caregiver and dentist approaches to improving oral care for children with autism. *Pediatric Dentistry, 41*(1), 4E–12E.

Taghizadeh, N., Heard, G., Davidson, A., Williams, K., & Story, D. (2019). The experiences of children with autism spectrum disorder, their caregivers and health care providers during day procedure: A mixed methods study. *Paediatric Anaesthesia, 29*(9), 927–937. https://doi.org/10.1111/pan.13689

Thomas, N., Blake, S., Morris, C., & Moles, D. R. (2018). Autism and primary care dentistry: Parents' experiences of taking children with autism or working diagnosis of autism for dental examinations. *International Journal of Paediatric Dentistry, 28*(2), 226–238. https://doi.org/10.1111/ipd.12345

Weir, E., Allison, C., & Baron-Cohen, S. (2022). Autistic adults have poorer quality healthcare and worse health based on self-report data. *Molecular Autism, 13*(1), 23. https://doi.org/10.1186/s13 229-022-00501-w

Chapter 4
Final Comments

This study had four objectives: first, to summarise the literature about the dental and medical experiences of autistics from the perspectives of autistics, their families, and professionals who treat autistics; second, to explain the barriers that autistic patients encounter while seeking medical and dental treatment and associated solutions to these barriers; third, to explain the limitations in the literature about the medical and dental experiences of autistics; and fourth, to provide strategies that can be used to help autistics participate in medical and dental examinations and procedures.

To achieve these objectives a search for relevant studies on PubMed was conducted during 12 November 2022. To ensure that the most relevant and contemporary studies were reviewed, only articles with the search terms in its title that were published five years before this study (i.e., all articles published after 12 November 2018) were examined. PubMed was searched because its repository of medical literature was deemed substantial and relevant. Despite its coverage not all studies that met the eligibility criteria were indexed on PubMed. Regardless of these limitations, the volume of studies retrieved for analysis was judged to be sufficient to answer the research questions.

An examination of the literature showed that within medical and dental environments some autistic patients have experienced a diverse range of challenges. For example, Weir and colleagues (2022) explained that most autistics in their study (n = 1003, 79.67%) claimed that the environment of the waiting room or office made them feel anxious. In another example, Mason and colleagues (2019) reported that of the six studies that they examined for their literature review four concluded that the healthcare system is too complex or inaccessible for autistics. Regarding dental care, Mirsky and colleagues (2021) reported that some autistic respondents in their study reported not enjoying the sensory sensation of small mental instruments scraping their teeth to remove plaque.

Based on the challenges identified in the literature, a series of strategies to help autistic patients have successful experiences in medical and dental clinics were formulated. For example, it was proposed that the sensory sensitivities that autistics encounter in clinical and dental settings could be mitigated. In another example, it was proposed that autistics could inform the doctor or dentist of their healthcare concerns by completing a form that explained such concerns. The strategies proposed at the end of Chaps. 2 and 3 were primarily intended for doctors and dentists.

The experiences in the reviewed literature are of value to dentists, medical doctors, those who research the autism spectrum, autistics, and parents who raise autistic children. Despite their value, it should be acknowledged that the results within these studies cannot be generalised to the broader autistic population because they were based on small sample sizes. Additionally, within several studies the participants did not need to prove that they were autistic or that they were parenting a child that was autistic. This lack of verification casts a doubt on the truthfulness of the results presented in these studies. On a more optimistic and final note, the limitations discovered in the examined literature gives researchers an opportunity to design studies in the future that will ultimately improve our understanding about the experiences of autistics in medical and dental clinics.

References

Mason, D., Ingham, B., Urbanowicz, A., Michael, C., Birtles, H., Woodbury-Smith, M., Brown, T., James, I., Scarlett, C., Nicolaidis, C., & Parr, J. R. (2019). A systematic review of what barriers and facilitators prevent and enable physical healthcare services access for autistic adults. *Journal of Autism and Developmental Disorders, 49*(8), 3387–3400. https://doi.org/10.1007/s10 803-019-04049-2

Mirsky, L. B., Rogo, E. J., & Gurenlian, J. R. (2021). Oral care experiences of young adults with autism spectrum disorder. *Journal of Dental Hygiene, 95*(4), 41–50.

Weir, E., Allison, C., & Baron-Cohen, S. (2022). Autistic adults have poorer quality healthcare and worse health based on self-report data. *Molecular Autism, 13*(1), 23. https://doi.org/10.1186/s13 229-022-00501-w

Appendices

Appendix 1.1: Summary of Studies About the Health Status of Autistic Adults

Authors	Diagnosis	Age of participants	Number of participants	Type of health	Title	Outcome
Baker and Richdale (2017)	ASD	18 and over	36	Physical and mental health	Examining the behavioural sleep-wake rhythm in adults with autism spectrum disorder and no comorbid intellectual disability	Participants completed a 14-day sleep-wake diary assessment. Results indicated that a higher proportion of adults with ASD met criteria for a circadian rhythm sleep-wake disorder compared to control adults. Delayed sleep-wake phase disorder was particularly common in adults with ASD. Results suggested that adults with ASD have sleep patterns associated with circadian rhythm disturbance; however, employment status and comorbid anxiety and/or depression appear to influence their sleep patterns

(continued)

G. Bennett, *Autistic People in Dental and Medical Clinics*, New Perspectives in Behavioral & Health Sciences, https://doi.org/10.1007/978-981-99-2359-5

(continued)

Authors	Diagnosis	Age of participants	Number of participants	Type of health	Title	Outcome
Baker et al. (2017)	ASD	18 and over	60	Physical health	Assessing the dim light melatonin onset in adults with autism spectrum disorder and no comorbid intellectual disability	Sixteen adults with ASD (ASD-Only), 12 adults with ASD medicated for comorbid diagnoses of anxiety and/or depression (ASD-Med), and 32 controls participated in the study. Overall, mean melatonin levels were lower in the ASD-Med group compared to that in the two other groups. Lastly, greater increases in melatonin in the hour prior to sleep were associated with greater sleep efficiency in the ASD groups
Buck et al. (2014)	ASD	18 and over	129	Mental health	Psychiatric comorbidity and medication use in adults with autism spectrum disorder	The comorbid psychiatric disorders and psychotropic medication use among adults with autism spectrum disorder (ASD) ascertained as children during a 1980s statewide Utah autism prevalence study were investigated. It was found that 56.6% met criteria for a current psychiatric disorder and 69.0% met lifetime criteria for a psychiatric disorder. Caregivers reported a psychiatric diagnosis in 34.1% of participants

(continued)

(continued)

Authors	Diagnosis	Age of participants	Number of participants	Type of health	Title	Outcome
Chen et al. (2016)	ASD	18–22	6122	Physical health	Risk of developing type 2 diabetes in adolescents and young adults with autism spectrum disorder: a nationwide longitudinal study	Adolescents and young adults with ASD had a higher risk of developing type 2 diabetes than those without ASD, after adjustment for demographic data, atypical antipsychotics use, and medical comorbidities. Sensitivity analyses after excluding first-year and first 3-year observation periods were consistent. Short-term and long-term use of atypical antipsychotics were associated with a higher likelihood of subsequent type 2 diabetes
Croen et al. (2015)	ASD	18 and over	1507 with ASD diagnoses 15,070 control group	Physical and mental health	Health status of adults on the ASD spectrum	The objective of this study was to describe the frequency of psychiatric and medical conditions among a large, diverse, insured population of adults with ASD in the United States. Adults with ASD had significantly increased rates of all major psychiatric disorders and medical conditions

(continued)

(continued)

Authors	Diagnosis	Age of participants	Number of participants	Type of health	Title	Outcome
Fortuna et al. (2016)	ASD	18–71	220	Physical and mental health	Health conditions and functional status in adults with autism: a cross-sectional evaluation	Adults with ASD have a high prevalence of seizure disorders and depression, but low rates of sexually transmitted infections, tobacco use, and alcohol misuse. Within our cohort, the majority of older adults with ASD required some assistance with activities of daily living
Gerber et al. (2017)	ASD	18–64	92	Physical and mental health	Brief report: factors influencing healthcare satisfaction in adults with autism spectrum disorder	Participants or their caregiver completed a survey about their experiences with primary care and specialty physicians. Participants under age 26 reported significantly higher levels of satisfaction than participants above age 26. They were more likely to live at home or have private health insurance indicating that a good family and community support will impact their healthcare satisfaction
Hamm and Yun (2019)	ASD	18–35	320	Physical and mental health	Influence of physical activity on the health-related quality of life of young adults with and without autism spectrum disorder	The presence of ASD significantly predicted overall health-related quality of life, the physical health domain, psychological domain, and the environment domain. Additionally, physical activity significantly predicted each domain and overall health-related quality of life regardless of the presence of autism spectrum disorder

(continued)

(continued)

Authors	Diagnosis	Age of participants	Number of participants	Type of health	Title	Outcome
Helverschou and Martinsen (2011)	ASD, intellectual disability	18 and over	62	Mental health	Anxiety in people diagnosed with autism and intellectual disability: recognition and phenomenology	The results indicated that anxiety can be recognised by symptoms similar to those in non-autistic individuals, but signs of physiological arousal seem difficult to recognise in this population. The results imply inclusion of general adjustment problems in order to identify individuals with anxiety problems by using a checklist. For diagnostic purposes, the use of an individual anxiety assessment seems indicated
Jones et al. (2016)	ASD	25-year study from children—mean age at follow-up 36	92	Physical health	A description of medical conditions in adults with autism spectrum disorder: a follow-up of the 1980s Utah/ UCLA autism epidemiologic study	The most common medical conditions were seizures, obesity, insomnia, and constipation. The median number of medical conditions per person was 11. Increased medical comorbidity was associated with female gender and obesity but not intellectual disability. Adults in this cohort of autism spectrum disorder first ascertained in the 1980s experience a high number of chronic medical conditions, regardless of intellectual ability

(continued)

(continued)

Authors	Diagnosis	Age of participants	Number of participants	Type of health	Title	Outcome
Khanna et al. (2014)	ASD	18 and over	291	Physical and mental health	Health-related quality of life and its determinants among adults with autism	Results revealed adults with ASD to have significantly lower physical and mental health-related quality of life (HRQOL) than their counterparts in the US population. Factors including social support and coping along with other sociodemographic and medial characteristics were identified as significant predictors of physical and mental HRQOL
Kohane et al. (2012)	ASD	Two groups 0–17 and 18–35 years	14,831 participants	Physical and mental health	The comorbidity burden of children and young adults with autism spectrum disorders	Used electronic health records to assess the comorbidity burden of ASD in under 18-year-olds to 18–34-year-olds. Three of the studied comorbidities increased significantly when comparing ages 0–17 vs. 18–34 with $P < 0.001$: schizophrenia (1.43% vs. 8.76%), diabetes mellitus type I (0.67% vs. 2.08%), and irritable bowel disorder (IBD; 0.68% vs. 1.99%); whereas sleeping disorders, bowel disorders (without IBD), and epilepsy did not change significantly

(continued)

(continued)

Authors	Diagnosis	Age of participants	Number of participants	Type of health	Title	Outcome
Lever and Geurts (2016)	ASD	19–79	247 ASD 208 control	Mental health	Psychiatric co-occurring symptoms and disorders in young, middle-aged, and older adults with autism spectrum disorder	Comparable to other psychiatric patients, adults with ASD showed high levels of symptoms and psychological distress over the adult lifespan. Over 65% of the adults with ASD meeting criteria for any lifetime mood or anxiety disorder also met criteria for the other co-occurring disorder
Limoges et al. (2013)	ASD	18–25	17	Physical health	Relationship between poor sleep and daytime cognitive performance in young adults with autism	Individuals with autism showed clear signs of poor sleep. Their performance differed from the controls in response speed but not in accuracy. Some signs reflecting the presence of poor sleep in adults with high-functioning autism correlate with various aspects of motor output on nonverbal performance tasks
Spain et al. (2016)	ASD	18 and over	50	Mental health	Social anxiety in adult males with autism spectrum disorders	Twenty-six participants (52%) endorsed levels of social anxiety that exceeded the suggested threshold for the disorder. Categorical and dimensional data analyses indicated that there were no relationships between SA symptoms, present state or childhood ASD symptom severity, or measures of socioemotional processing in this sample

(continued)

(continued)

Authors	Diagnosis	Age of participants	Number of participants	Type of health	Title	Outcome
Totsika et al. (2010)	ASD, intellectual disability	50 years or older	46	Physical and mental health	Behaviour problems, psychiatric symptoms, and quality of life for older adults with intellectual disability with and without autism	Intellectual disability (ID) and the triad of impairments characteristic of ASD were compared to peers with ID only, and younger adults with ASD and ID. Older adults with ASD did not differ from those with ID in terms of behaviour problems, psychiatric disorder, and quality of life. Any differences in the skills of adults with ASD were associated with decreased adaptive skills and not the presence of ASD per se
Tyler et al. (2011)	ASD	18 and over	108	Physical and mental health	Chronic disease risks in young adults with autism spectrum disorder: forewarned is forearmed	Used electronic health record (EHR) analysis to examine prevalent and future health risks of persons with disabilities. Rates of chronic disease included 34.9% for obesity, 31.5% for hyperlipidaemia, and 19.4% for hypertension. Compared with a control, adults with ASD were more likely to be diagnosed with hyperlipidaemia. Without intervention, they appear to be at risk for developing diabetes, coronary heart disease, and cancer by midlife

(continued)

(continued)

Authors	Diagnosis	Age of participants	Number of participants	Type of health	Title	Outcome
Vogan et al. (2017)	ASD	18–61 years	40	Physical and mental health	Tracking health care service use and the experiences of adults with autism spectrum disorder	Examined a diverse range of medical and mental health services and supports, as well as adults' personal experiences accessing and using these services, and barriers to service use. Results indicated that beyond a family doctor, the most commonly used services were dentistry and psychiatry. Individuals who had medical problems experienced significantly more barriers to service use than those who did not
Wakeford et al. (2015)	ASD, epilepsy	18 and over	163	Physical health	Autistic characteristics in adults with epilepsy and perceived seizure activity	These results suggested that adults with epilepsy have higher autistic characteristics measured by the social responsiveness scale, while sameness behaviours remain unimpaired. The autistic characteristics measured by the social responsiveness scale were reported by adults with epilepsy to be more severe during their mild seizure activity

(continued)

(continued)

Authors	Diagnosis	Age of participants	Number of participants	Type of health	Title	Outcome
Wallace et al. (2016)	ASD	18 and over	35	Mental health	Real-world executive functions in adults with autism spectrum disorder: profiles of impairment and associations with adaptive functioning and comorbid anxiety and depression	A variable executive functions profile was found with prominent deficits occurring in flexibility and metacognition. Flexibility problems were associated with anxiety-related symptoms, while metacognition difficulties were associated with depression symptoms and impaired adaptive functioning. These are predictors of broader functioning and therefore remain an important treatment target among adults with ASD
Westwood et al. (2017)	ASD	18 and over	60	Physical and mental health	Clinical evaluation of autistic symptoms in women with anorexia nervosa	Fourteen women (23.3%) scored above clinical cutoff for ASD on the ADOS-2. Only eight of these women displayed repetitive or restrictive behaviours, while all 14 had difficulties with social affect. Elevated ASD symptoms were associated with increased alexithymia and obsessive-compulsive symptoms, but not specific eating disorder pathology

Source Forde, J., Bonilla, P. M., Mannion, A., Coyne, R., Haverty, R., & Leader, G. (2022). Health status of adults with autism spectrum disorder. *Review Journal of Autism and Developmental Disorders, 9*(3), 427–437. https://doi.org/10.1007/s40489-021-00267-6

References

Baker, E., & Richdale, A. (2017). Examining the behavioural sleep-wake rhythm in adults with autism spectrum disorder and no comorbid intellectual disability. *Journal of Autism and Developmental Disorders, 47*(4), 1207–1222. https://doi.org/10.1007/s10803-017-3042-3

Baker, E., Richdale, A., Hazi, A., & Prendergast, L. (2017). Assessing the dim light melatonin onset in adults with autism spectrum disorder and no comorbid intellectual disability. *Journal of Autism and Developmental Disorders, 47*(7), 2120–2137. https://doi.org/10.1007/s10803-017-3122-4

Buck, T. R., Viskochil, J., Farley, M., Coon, H., McMahon, W. M., Morgan, J., & Bilder, D. A. (2014). Psychiatric comorbidity and medication use in adults with autism spectrum disorder. *Journal of Autism and Developmental Disorders, 44*(12), 3063–3071. https://doi.org/10.1007/s10803-014-2170-2

Chen, M. H., Lan, W. H., Hsu, J. W., Huang, K. L., Su, T. P., Li, C. T., ... & Bai, Y. M. (2016). Risk of developing type 2 diabetes in adolescents and young adults with autism spectrum disorder: A nationwide longitudinal study. *Diabetes Care, 39*(5), 788–793. https://doi.org/10.2337/dc15-1807

Croen, L., Zerbo, O., Qian, Y., Massolo, M., Rich, S., Sidney, S., & Kripke, C. (2015). The health status of adults on the autism spectrum. *Autism: The International Journal of Research and Practice, 19*(7), 814–823. https://doi.org/10.1177/1362361315577517

Fortuna, R., Robinson, L., Smith, T., Meccarello, J., Bullen, B., Nobis, K., & Davidson, P. (2016). Health conditions and functional status in adults with autism: A cross-sectional evaluation. *Journal of General Internal Medicine, 31*(1), 77–84. https://doi.org/10.1007/s11606-015-3509-x

Gerber, A. H., McCormick, C. E., Levine, T. P., Morrow, E. M., Anders, T. F., & Sheinkopf, S. J. (2017). Brief report: Factors influencing healthcare satisfaction in adults with autism spectrum disorder. *Journal of Autism and Developmental Disorders, 47*(6), 1896–1903. https://doi.org/10.1007/s10803-017-3087-3

Hamm, J., & Yun, J. (2019). Influence of physical activity on the health-related quality of life of young adults with and without autism spectrum disorder. *Disability and Rehabilitation, 41*(7), 763–769. https://doi.org/10.1080/09638288.2017.1408708

Helverschou, S., & Martinsen, H. (2011). Anxiety in people diagnosed with autism and intellectual disability: Recognition and phenomenology. *Research in Autism Spectrum Disorders, 5*(1), 377–387. https://doi.org/10.1016/j.rasd.2010.05.003

Jones, K., Cottle, K., Bakian, A., Farley, M., Bilder, D., Coon, H., & McMahon, W. (2016). A description of medical conditions in adults with autism spectrum disorder: A follow-up of the 1980s Utah/UCLA autism epidemiologic study. *Autism: The International Journal of Research and Practice, 20*(5), 551–561. https://doi.org/10.1177/1362361315594798

Khanna, R., Jariwala-Parikh, K., West-Strum, D., & Mahabaleshwarkar, R. (2014). Health-related quality of life and its determinants among adults with autism. *Research in Autism Spectrum Disorders, 8*(3), 157–167. https://doi.org/10.1016/j.rasd.2013.11.003

Kohane, I. S., McMurry, A., Weber, G., MacFadden, D., Rappaport, L., Kunkel, L., Bickel, J., Wattanasin, N., Spence, S., Murphy, S., & Churchill, S. (2012). The co-morbidity burden of children and young adults with autism spectrum disorders. *PLoS One, 7*(4), e33224. https://doi.org/10.1371/journal.pone.0033224

Lever, A. G., & Geurts, H. M. (2016). Psychiatric co-occurring symptoms and disorders in young, middle-aged, and older adults with autism spectrum disorder. *Journal of Autism and Developmental Disorders, 46*(6), 1916–1930. https://doi.org/10.1007/s10803-016-2722-8

Limoges, É., Bolduc, C., Berthiaume, C., Mottron, L., & Godbout, R. (2013). Relationship between poor sleep and daytime cognitive performance in young adults with autism. *Research in Developmental Disabilities, 34*(4), 1322–1335. https://doi.org/10.1016/j.ridd.2013.01.013

Spain, D., Happé, F., Johnston, P., Campbell, M., Sin, J., Daly, E., Ecker, C., Anson, M., Chaplin, E., Glaser, K., Mendez, A., Lovell, K., & Murphy, D. (2016). Social anxiety in adult males with autism spectrum disorders. *Research in Autism Spectrum Disorders, 32*, 13–23. https://doi.org/10.1016/j.rasd.2016.08.002

Totsika, V., Felce, D., Kerr, M., & Hastings, R. (2010). Behavior problems, psychiatric symptoms, and quality of life for older adults with intellectual disability with and without autism. *Journal of Autism and Developmental Disorders, 40*(10), 1171–1178. https://doi.org/10.1007/s10803-010-0975-1

Tyler, C., Schramm, S., Karafa, M., Tang, A., & Jain, A. (2011). Chronic disease risks in young adults with autism spectrum disorder: Forewarned is forearmed. *American Journal on Intellectual and Developmental Disabilities, 116*(5), 371–380. https://doi.org/10.1352/1944-7558-116.5.371

Vogan, V., Lake, J., Tint, A., Weiss, J., & Lunsky, Y. (2017). Tracking health care service use and the experiences of adults with autism spectrum disorder without intellectual disability: A longitudinal study of service rates, barriers and satisfaction. *Disability and Health Journal, 10*(2), 264–270. https://doi.org/10.1016/j.dhjo.2016.11.002

Wakeford, S., Hinvest, N., Ring, H., & Brosnan, M. (2015). Autistic characteristics in adults with epilepsy and perceived seizure activity. *Epilepsy & Behavior, 52*, 244–250. https://doi.org/10.1016/j.yebeh.2015.08.031

Wallace, G., Kenworthy, L., Pugliese, C., Popal, H., White, E., Brodsky, E., & Martin, A. (2016). Real-world executive functions in adults with autism spectrum disorder: Profiles of impairment and associations with adaptive functioning and co-morbid anxiety and depression. *Journal of Autism and Developmental Disorders, 46*(3), 1071–1083. https://doi.org/10.1007/s10803-015-2655-7

Westwood, H., Mandy, W., & Tchanturia, K. (2017). Clinical evaluation of *autistic* symptoms in women with anorexia nervosa. *Molecular Autism, 8*(12). https://doi.org/10.1186/s13229-017-0128-x

Appendix 1.2: Evaluation Form for Studies Selected for Examination

Criteria	Answer
Reference for the citation	
Is this article distributed under the terms of the Creative Commons Attribution 4.0 International License (http://creativecommons.org/licenses/by/4.0/), *which permits unrestricted use, distribution, and reproduction in any medium, provided you give appropriate credit to the original author(s) and the source, provide a link to the Creative Commons license, and indicate if changes were made?*	Yes No
Sample size	
Limitations of the study	
Quotes	

Appendix 1.3: Dataset

PubMed ID	First author	Article title	Citation information	Reason why the citation was either included or excluded
36357551	da Silva Moro J	Efficacy of the Video Modeling Technique as a Facilitator of Non-invasive Dental Care in Autistic Children: Randomized Clinical Trial	*J Autism Dev Disord.* 2022 Nov 10. https://doi.org/10.1007/s10803-022-05820-8. Online ahead of print	EXCLUDED—Article did not answer any research questions
36354158[†]	Sherriff A	Child oral health and preventive dental service access among children with intellectual disabilities, autism and other educational additional support needs: A population-based record linkage cohort study	*Community Dent Oral Epidemiol.* 2022 Nov 10. https://doi.org/10.1111/cdoe.12805. Online ahead of print	EXCLUDED—Article did not answer any research questions
36271894	Junnarkar VS	Qualitative study on barriers and coping strategies for dental care in autistic children: Parents' perspective	*Int J Paediatr Dent.* 2022 Oct 22. https://doi.org/10.1111/ipd.13035. Online ahead of print	INCLUDED—Citation described barriers to dental care for autistic children through the experiences and opinions of their parents
36238091	Zerman N	Insights on dental care management and prevention in children with autism spectrum disorder (ASD). What is new?	*Front Oral Health.* 2022 Sep 27;3:998831. https://doi.org/10.3389/froh.2022.998831. eCollection 2022	EXCLUDED—Article did not answer any research questions
36224087	Cenzon KF	Use of a Simulated-Virtual Training Module to Improve Dental Hygiene Students' Self-Reported Knowledge, Attitudes, and Confidence in Providing Care to Children with Autism Spectrum Disorder: A pilot study	*J Dent Hyg.* 2022 Oct;96(5):42–51	EXCLUDED—Article did not answer any research questions

(continued)

(continued)

PubMed ID	First author	Article title	Citation information	Reason why the citation was either included or excluded
36120282[†]	Verma A	Assessment of Parental Perceptions of Socio-Psychological Factors, Unmet Dental Needs, and Barriers to Utilise Oral Health Care in Autistic Children	*Cureus.* 2022 Aug 12;14(8):e27950. https://doi.org/10.7759/cureus.27950. eCollection 2022 Aug	EXCLUDED—Article did not answer any research questions
35799335	Cai J	Parents' Perceptions Regarding the Effectiveness of Dental Desensitization for Children with Autism Spectrum Disorder	*Pediatr Dent.* 2022 May 15;44(3):192–197	EXCLUDED—Article did not answer any research questions
35718919	Azimi S	Dental procedures in children with or without intellectual disability and autism spectrum disorder in a hospital setting	*Aust Dent J.* 2022 Jun 19. https://doi.org/10.1111/adj.12927. Online ahead of print	EXCLUDED—Article did not answer any research questions
35716111[†]	Erwin J	Factors influencing oral health behaviours, access and delivery of dental care for autistic children and adolescents: A mixed-methods systematic review	*Health Expect.* 2022 Aug;25(4):1269–1318. https://doi.org/10.1111/hex.13544. Epub 2022 Jun 18	INCLUDED—This study aimed to gather evidence on the factors that influence oral health behaviours, access to, and delivery of dental care for autistic youth
35703705	Paula VAC	Responsiveness of the B-ECOHIS to detect changes in OHRQoL following dental treatment of children with autism spectrum disorder	*Braz Oral Res.* 2022 Jun 10:36:e079. https://doi.org/10.1590/1807-3107bor-2022.vol36.0079. eCollection 2022	EXCLUDED—Article did not answer any research questions

(continued)

(continued)

PubMed ID	First author	Article title	Citation information	Reason why the citation was either included or excluded
35654391	Alvares GA	Dental care experiences and clinical phenotypes in children on the autism spectrum	*Spec Care Dentist*. 2022 Jun 2. https://doi.org/10.1111/scd.12746. Online ahead of print	INCLUDED—This study investigated parental reports of oral health and dental service needs of children diagnosed with autism and explored relationships with clinical phenotypes
35645511	Babu NV	Comparative Analysis of the Status of Dental Caries and Selected Salivary Electrolytes in Children with Autism	*Int J Clin Pediatr Dent*. 2022;15(Suppl 2):S242–S246. https://doi.org/10.5005/jp-journals-10005-2153	EXCLUDED—Article did not answer any research questions
35636432	McNeil R	Are adults with autism receiving regular preventive dental services?	*Spec Care Dentist*. 2022 May 30. https://doi.org/10.1111/scd.12738. Online ahead of print	EXCLUDED—Article did not answer any research questions
35526843[†]	Aljubour A	Effect of Culturally Adapted Dental Visual Aids on Oral Hygiene Status during Dental Visits in Children with Autism Spectrum Disorder: A Randomized Clinical Trial	*Children (Basel)*. 2022 May 5;9(5):666. https://doi.org/10.3390/children9050666	EXCLUDED—Article did not answer any research questions
35589819	Balian A	Long-term caries prevention of dental sealants and fluoride varnish in children with autism spectrum disorders: a retrospective cohort study	*Sci Rep*. 2022 May 19;12(1):8478. https://doi.org/10.1038/s41598-022-12176-7	EXCLUDED—Article did not answer any research questions
35579049	Mac Giolla Phadraig C	Promoting openness to autism amongst dental care professional students	*Eur J Dent Educ*. 2022 May 17. https://doi.org/10.1111/eje.12821. Online ahead of print	EXCLUDED—Article did not answer any research questions

(continued)

(continued)

PubMed ID	First author	Article title	Citation information	Reason why the citation was either included or excluded
35561086	Junnarkar VS	Occupational and speech therapists' perceptions of their role in dental care for children with autism spectrum disorder: A qualitative exploration	*Int J Paediatr Dent*. 2022 Nov;32(6):865–876. https://doi.org/10.1111/ipd.13009. Epub 2022 May 27	EXCLUDED—Article did not answer any research questions
35524299	AlBhaisi IN	Effectiveness of psychological techniques in dental management for children with autism spectrum disorder: a systematic literature review	*BMC Oral Health*. 2022 May 6;22(1):162. https://doi.org/10.1186/s12903-022-02200-7	EXCLUDED—This paper was a literature review
35463526	Park Y	Dental Anxiety in Children With Autism Spectrum Disorder: Understanding Frequency and Associated Variables	*Front Psychiatry*. 2022 Apr 7:13:838557. https://doi.org/10.3389/fpsyt.2022.838557. eCollection 2022	EXCLUDED—Article did not answer any research questions
35327765	Fallea A	Sensory-Adapted Dental Environment for the Treatment of Patients with Autism Spectrum Disorder	*Children (Basel)*. 2022 Mar 10;9(3):393. https://doi.org/10.3390/children9030393	INCLUDED—Article answered the research question
35248005†	Piraneh H	Oral health and dental caries experience among students aged 7–15 years old with autism spectrum disorders in Tehran, Iran	*BMC Pediatr*. 2022 Mar 5;22(1):116. https://doi.org/10.1186/s12887-022-03178-5	EXCLUDED—Article did not answer any research questions
35211746	Fenning RM	Parent Training for Dental Care in Underserved Children With Autism: A Randomized Controlled Trial	*Pediatrics*. 2022 May 1;149(5):e2021050691. https://doi.org/10.1542/peds.2021-050691	EXCLUDED—Article did not answer any research questions

(continued)

(continued)

PubMed ID	First author	Article title	Citation information	Reason why the citation was either included or excluded
35068893[†]	AlHumaid J	Dental experiences related to oral care of children with autism spectrum disorders in Saudi Arabia: A literature review	*Saudi Dent J.* 2022 Jan;34(1):1–10. https://doi.org/10.1016/j.sdentj.2021.09.023. Epub 2021 Sep 27	INCLUDED—This study is a review of the published literature related to dental experiences of autistic children in Saudi Arabia
35048025	Tran J	An Investigation of the Long and Short Term Behavioral Effects of General Anesthesia on Pediatric Dental Patients With Autism	*Front Oral Health.* 2021 Aug 17;2:679946. https://doi.org/10.3389/froh.2021.679946. eCollection 2021	EXCLUDED—Article did not answer any research questions
34897755	Azevedo Machado B	Fear, changes in routine and dental care for children and adolescents with autism spectrum disorder in the COVID-19 pandemic: A survey with Brazilian parents	*Spec Care Dentist.* 2022 Jul;42(4):352–360. https://doi.org/10.1111/scd.12683. Epub 2021 Dec 13	EXCLUDED—Article did not answer any research questions
34886072[†]	Erwin J	Factors Influencing Oral Health Behaviours, Access and Provision of Dental Care for Autistic Children and Adolescents in Countries with a Very High Human Development Index: Protocol for a Mixed Methods Systematic Review	*Int J Environ Res Public Health.* 2021 Nov 24;18(23):12346. https://doi.org/10.3390/ije rph182312346	EXCLUDED—This study was a protocol

(continued)

(continued)

PubMed ID	First author	Article title	Citation information	Reason why the citation was either included or excluded
34693784	Parry JA	Dental Visits for Autistic Children: A Qualitative Focus Group Study of Parental Perceptions	*JDR Clin Trans Res.* 2021 Oct 23:23800844211049404. https://doi.org/10.1177/23800844211049404. Online ahead of print	INCLUDED—This study aimed to examine parental perceptions of difficulties associated with dental attendance and oral care for autistic children and young adults, to highlight reported challenges and potential adaptations, and to identify interventions that will encourage positive experiences of dental attendance
34582574	McMillion A	UK-based specialist dental professionals' experiences of working with autistic patients	*Spec Care Dentist.* 2022 Mar;42(2):120–136. https://doi.org/10.1111/scd.12653. Epub 2021 Sep 28	INCLUDED—The aim of this study was to investigate the strategies UK-based dental professionals' use when working with autistic patients
34540992	Marra PM	Dental Trauma in Children with Autistic Disorder: A Retrospective Study	*Biomed Res Int.* 2021 Sep 8:2021:3125251. https://doi.org/10.1155/2021/3125251. eCollection 2021	EXCLUDED—Article did not answer any research questions
34501850	Hong SJ	A Digital Fabrication of Dental Prosthesis for Preventing Self-Injurious Behavior Related to Autism Spectrum Disorder: A Case Report	*Int J Environ Res Public Health.* 2021 Sep 2;18(17):9249. https://doi.org/10.3390/ijerph18179249	EXCLUDED—Article did not answer any research questions

(continued)

(continued)

PubMed ID	First author	Article title	Citation information	Reason why the citation was either included or excluded
34490770	Schreuder S	Mental disorders in the dental practice. Autism spectrum disorder	*Ned Tijdschr Tandheelkd.* 2021 Sep;128(9):451–455. https://doi.org/10.5177/ntvt.2021.09.21060	EXCLUDED—This article is published in Dutch
34467849	Gandhi R	Association Between Autism Spectrum Disorder and Dental Anomalies of the Permanent Dentition	*Pediatr Dent.* 2021 Jul 15;43(4):307–312	EXCLUDED—Article did not answer any research questions
34148478	Azimi S	Factors associated with dental hospitalisations in children with intellectual disability or autism spectrum disorder: a Western Australian population-based retrospective cohort study	*Disabil Rehabil.* 2022 Sep;44(19):5495–5503. https://doi.org/10.1080/09638288.2021.193 6662. Epub 2021 Jun 19	EXCLUDED—Article did not answer any research questions
34043844[†]	de Almeida JS	Impact of dental treatment on the oral health-related quality of life of children and adolescents with Autism Spectrum Disorder	*Spec Care Dentist.* 2021 Nov;41(6):658–669. https://doi.org/10.1111/scd.12618. Epub 2021 May 27	EXCLUDED—Article did not answer any research questions
33852747	Dumbuya A	Types of dental procedures provided to adults with autism spectrum condition: A descriptive study	*Spec Care Dentist.* 2021 Sep;41(5):553–558. https://doi.org/10.1111/scd.12596. Epub 2021 Apr 14	EXCLUDED—Article did not answer any research questions
33772132	Thomas N	Dental disease risk in children with autism: a meta-analysis	*Evid Based Dent.* 2021 Jan;22(1):34–35. https://doi.org/10.1038/s41432-021-0165-3	EXCLUDED—Article did not answer any research questions

(continued)

(continued)

PubMed ID	First author	Article title	Citation information	Reason why the citation was either included or excluded
33682191	McMillion A	Dental experiences of a group of autistic adults based in the United Kingdom	*Spec Care Dentist*. 2021 Jul;41(4):474–488. https://doi.org/10.1111/scd.12583. Epub 2021 Mar 7	INCLUDED—The current study investigated autistic adults' dental experiences in the UK
33573642[†]	Alshatrat SM	Oral health knowledge and dental behavior among individuals with autism in Jordan: a case–control study	*BMC Oral Health*. 2021 Feb 11;21(1):62. https://doi.org/10.1186/s12903-021-01423-4	EXCLUDED—Article did not answer any research questions
33559018	Parry JA	Brief Report: Analysis of Dental Treatment Provided Under General Anaesthesia for Children and Young Adults with Autistic Spectrum Disorder and Identification of Challenges for Dental Services	*J Autism Dev Disord*. 2021 Dec;51(12):4698–4703. https://doi.org/10.1007/s10803-021-04898-w. Epub 2021 Feb 8	EXCLUDED—Article did not answer any research questions
33477719[†]	Balian A	Is Visual Pedagogy Effective in Improving Cooperation Towards Oral Hygiene and Dental Care in Children with Autism Spectrum Disorder? A Systematic Review and Meta-Analysis	*Int J Environ Res Public Health*. 2021 Jan 18;18(2):789. https://doi.org/10.3390/ijerph18020789	EXCLUDED—Article did not answer any research questions
33382440	Kind LS	Parents' satisfaction on dental care of Dutch children with Autism Spectrum Disorder	*Eur Arch Paediatr Dent*. 2021 Jun;22(3):491–496. https://doi.org/10.1007/s40368-020-00586-y. Epub 2021 Jun 18	INCLUDED—To assess if autistic children in Holland regularly visit a dentist and to evaluate a parent's satisfaction on the care provided

(continued)

(continued)

PubMed ID	First author	Article title	Citation information	Reason why the citation was either included or excluded
33350958[†]	Spivack E	Medical comorbidities associated with autism spectrum disorder and their impact on dental care	*Gen Dent.* 2021 Jan–Feb;69(1):62–68	EXCLUDED—Article did not answer any research questions
33245441	Alshihri AA	Correction to: Barriers to Professional Dental Care among Children with Autism Spectrum Disorder	*J Autism Dev Disord.* 2021 Aug;51(8):2995. https://doi.org/10.1007/s10803-020-04791-y. Epub 2020 Nov 27	EXCLUDED—This is a correction of a previous article
33224533	Chybicki D	Computer-Controlled Local Anesthesia Complication: Surgical Retrieval of a Broken Dental Needle in Noncooperative Autistic Paediatric Patient	*Case Rep Dent.* 2020 Nov 10:2020:6686736. https://doi.org/10.1155/2020/6686736. eCollection 2020	EXCLUDED—Article did not answer any research questions
33203140	Endres D	New Cav1.2 Channelopathy with High-Functioning Autism, Affective Disorder, Severe Dental Enamel Defects, a Short QT Interval, and a Novel CACNA1C Loss-Of-Function Mutation	*Int J Mol Sci.* 2020 Nov 15:21(22):8611. https://doi.org/10.3390/ijms21228611	EXCLUDED—Article did not answer any research questions
33089446	Alshihri AA	Barriers to Professional Dental Care among Children with Autism Spectrum Disorder	*J Autism Dev Disord.* 2021 Aug;51(8):2988–2994. https://doi.org/10.1007/s10803-020-04759-y. Epub 2020 Oct 21	INCLUDED—This study answered the research question
32880788	Logrieco MGM	What Happens at a Dental Surgery When the Patient is a Child with Autism Spectrum Disorder? An Italian Study	*J Autism Dev Disord.* 2021 Jun;51(6):1939–1952. https://doi.org/10.1007/s10803-020-04684-0	INCLUDED—Article answered the research question

(continued)

(continued)

PubMed ID	First author	Article title	Citation information	Reason why the citation was either included or excluded
32878399	Wu XR	Analysis of caries experience and the dental treatments under general anesthesia in 103 cases of children with autism spectrum disorders	*Zhonghua Kou Qiang Yi Xue Za Zhi.* 2020 Sep 9;55(9):639–646. https://doi.org/10.3760/cma.j.cn112144-20200321-00163	EXCLUDED—This study was published in Chinese
32831836	Alshatrat SM	Dental Service Utilization and Barriers to Dental Care for Individuals with Autism Spectrum Disorder in Jordan: A Case–Control Study	*Int J Dent.* 2020 Aug 3;2020:3035463. https://doi.org/10.1155/2020/3035463. eCollection 2020	INCLUDED—The aim of this study was to examine the use of dental services in autistic individuals in Jordan and identify barriers that affect their access to dental care in comparison with non-autistic individuals
32788003	Taneja N	Caregivers' Barriers to Dental Care for Children with Autism Spectrum Disorder	*J Dent Child (Chic).* 2020 May 15;87(2):98–102	INCLUDED—This study investigated caregivers' perspective on barriers to dental care for autistic children *THIS STUDY COULD NOT BE ACCESSED*
32728144	Kurek M	Disturbances in primary dental enamel in Polish autistic children	*Sci Rep.* 2020 Jul 29;10(1):12751. https://doi.org/10.1038/s41598-020-69642-3	EXCLUDED—Article did not answer any research questions
32664704	Narzisi A	"Mom Let's Go to the Dentist!" Preliminary Feasibility of a Tailored Dental Intervention for Children with Autism Spectrum Disorder in the Italian Public Health Service	*Brain Sci.* 2020 Jul 12;10(7):444. https://doi.org/10.3390/brainsci10070444	INCLUDED—Article answered the research question

(continued)

(continued)

PubMed ID	First author	Article title	Citation information	Reason why the citation was either included or excluded
32489813	Sultan A	Co-morbidity of down syndrome with autism spectrum disorder: Dental implications	*J Oral Biol Craniofac Res.* 2020 Apr–Jun;10(2):146–148. https://doi.org/10.1016/j.jobcr.2020.03.014. Epub 2020 Apr 11	EXCLUDED—Article did not answer any research questions
32308318	Penmetsa C	Role of Dental Discomfort Questionnaire-Based Approach in Recognition of Symptomatic Expressions Due to Dental Pain in Children with Autism Spectrum Disorders	*Contemp Clin Dent.* 2019 Jul–Sep;10(3):446–451. https://doi.org/10.4103/ccd.ccd_728_18	EXCLUDED—Article did not answer any research questions
32140982[†]	Naidoo M	A Dental Communication Board as an Oral Care Tool for Children with Autism Spectrum Disorder	*J Autism Dev Disord.* 2020 Nov;50(11):3831–3843. https://doi.org/10.1007/s10803-020-04436-0	EXCLUDED—Article did not answer any research questions.
32112232	Fenning RM	Access to Dental Visits and Correlates of Preventive Dental Care in Children with Autism Spectrum Disorder	*J Autism Dev Disord.* 2020 Oct;50(10):3739–3747. https://doi.org/10.1007/s10803-020-04420-8	EXCLUDED—Article did not answer any research questions
32008179	Zhang Y	Dental Caries Status in Autistic Children: A Meta-analysis	*J Autism Dev Disord.* 2020 Apr;50(4):1249–1257. https://doi.org/10.1007/s10803-019-04256-x	EXCLUDED—Article did not answer any research questions
31882559	Dailey JC	Autism Spectrum Disorder: Techniques for dental radiographic examinations	*J Dent Hyg.* 2019 Dec;93(6):35–41	EXCLUDED—Article did not answer any research questions
31648672	Yost Q	Children with Autism Spectrum Disorder Are Able to Maintain Dental Skills: A Two-Year Case Review of Desensitization Treatment	*Pediatr Dent.* 2019 Sep 15;41(5):397–403	EXCLUDED—Article did not answer any research questions

(continued)

(continued)

PubMed ID	First author	Article title	Citation information	Reason why the citation was either included or excluded
31562451	Eades D	UK dental professionals' knowledge, experience and confidence when treating patients on the autism spectrum	*Br Dent J.* 2019 Sep;227(6):504–510. https://doi.org/10.1038/s41415-019-0786-5	INCLUDED—Article answered the research question
31552917	Hariyani N	Factors influencing the severity of dental caries among Indonesian children with autism spectrum disorder - a pilot study	*Clin Cosmet Investig Dent.* 2019 Jul 29;11:227–233. https://doi.org/10.2147/CCIDE.S205041. eCollection 2019	EXCLUDED—Article did not answer any research questions
31490715	Burgette JM	Association between Autism Spectrum Disorder and Caregiver-Reported Dental Caries in Children	*JDR Clin Trans Res.* 2020 Jul;5(3):254–261. https://doi.org/10.1177/2380084419875441. Epub 2019 Sep 6	EXCLUDED—Article did not answer any research questions
31332568	Mangione F	Autistic patients: a retrospective study on their dental needs and the behavioural approach	*Clin Oral Investig.* 2020 May;24(5):1677–1685. https://doi.org/10.1007/s00784-019-03023-7. Epub 2019 Jul 22	EXCLUDED—Article did not answer any research questions
31317073[†]	Lai J	Designing a program evaluation for a medical-dental service for adults with autism and intellectual disabilities using the RE-AIM framework	*Learn Health Syst.* 2019 Apr 1;3(3):e10192. https://doi.org/10.1002/lrh2.10192. eCollection 2019 Jul	EXCLUDED—Article did not answer any research questions
30969385	Limeres J	Brief Report: Estimating the Dental Age of Children with Autism Spectrum Disorders	*J Autism Dev Disord.* 2019 Jun;49(6):2612–2617. https://doi.org/10.1007/s10803-019-04007-y	EXCLUDED—Article did not answer any research questions
30875300	El-Maghraby A	Treating dental patients with autism spectrum disorder	*Gen Dent.* 2019 Mar–Apr;67(2):14-16	EXCLUDED—Article did not answer any research questions

(continued)

(continued)

PubMed ID	First author	Article title	Citation information	Reason why the citation was either included or excluded
30592319	Holt S	Parent-reported experience of using a real-time text messaging service for dental appointments for children and young people with autism spectrum conditions: A pilot study	*Spec Care Dentist*. 2019 Mar;39(2):84–88. https://doi.org/10.1111/scd.12347. Epub 2018 Dec 28	EXCLUDED—Article did not answer any research questions
30190742	Al-Sehaibany FS	Occurrence of traumatic dental injuries among preschool children with Autism Spectrum Disorder	*Pak J Med Sci*. 2018 Jul–Aug;34(4):859–863. https://doi.org/10.12669/pjms.344.15681	EXCLUDED—Article did not answer any research questions
30136115[†]	Du RY	Oral Health Behaviours of Preschool Children with Autism Spectrum Disorders and Their Barriers to Dental Care	*J Autism Dev Disord*. 2019 Feb;49(2):453–459. https://doi.org/10.1007/s10803-018-3708-5	INCLUDED—This study compared oral health behaviours and barriers to dental care among preschool autistic and non-autistic children and evaluated dental knowledge and attitudes of their parents
30131645	Chandrashekhar S	Management of Autistic Patients in Dental Office: A Clinical Update	*Int J Clin Pediatr Dent*. 2018 May–Jun;11(3):219–227. https://doi.org/10.5005/jp-journals-10005-1515. Epub 2018 Jun 1	EXCLUDED—Article did not answer any research questions
29643711	Chang KC	Dental utilization and expenditures by children and adolescents with autism spectrum disorders: A population-based cohort study	*Ci Ji Yi Xue Za Zhi*. 2018 Jan–Mar;30(1):15–19. https://doi.org/10.4103/tcmj.tcmj_185_17	EXCLUDED—Article did not answer any research questions

(continued)

(continued)

PubMed ID	First author	Article title	Citation information	Reason why the citation was either included or excluded
29482677	Zink AG	Communication Application for Use During the First Dental Visit for Children and Adolescents with Autism Spectrum Disorders	*Pediatr Dent.* 2018 Jan 1;40(1):18–22	INCLUDED—Citation described a strategy to help autistics undergo dental examinations *THIS STUDY COULD NOT BE ACCESSED*
29197446	Tounsi A	Children With Autism Spectrum Disorders can be Successfully Examined Using Dental Desensitization	*J Evid Based Dent Pract.* 2017 Dec;17(4):414–415. https://doi.org/10.1016/j.jebdp.2017.10.007. Epub 2017 Oct 16	EXCLUDED—This is an academic commentary
29073339	Thomas N	Autism and primary care dentistry: parents' experiences of taking children with autism or working diagnosis of autism for dental examinations	*Int J Paediatr Dent.* 2018 Mar;28(2):226–238. https://doi.org/10.1111/ipd.12345. Epub 2017 Oct 26	INCLUDED—To gather dental experiences of UK parents of autistic children or working diagnosis of autism and explore how they feel primary care dental services can be improved
36183860	Penna HM	Comparison between oral midazolam versus oral ketamine plus midazolam as preanesthetic medication in autism spectrum disorder: double-blind randomized clinical trial	*Braz J Anesthesiol.* 2022 Sep 29:S0104-0014(22)00124-5. https://doi.org/10.1016/j.bjane.2022.09.003. Online ahead of print	EXCLUDED—Article did not answer any research questions
36138725	Como DH	Oral Care Knowledge, Attitudes, and Practices of Black/African American Caregivers of Autistic Children and Non-Autistic Children	*Children (Basel).* 2022 Sep 19;9(9):1417. https://doi.org/10.3390/children9091417	EXCLUDED—Article did not answer any research questions

(continued)

(continued)

PubMed ID	First author	Article title	Citation information	Reason why the citation was either included or excluded
36110675	Pawar M	Manual and Powered Toothbrushing Effectiveness on Autistic Children's Oral Hygiene Status	*J Pharm Bioallied Sci.* 2022 Jul;14(Suppl 1):S837-S840. https://doi.org/10.4103/jpbs.jpbs_15_22. Epub 2022 Jul 13	EXCLUDED—Article did not answer any research questions
36071687	Maes P	Describing (pre)linguistic oral productions in 3- to 5-year-old autistic children: A cluster analysis	*Autism.* 2022 Sep 7:13623613221122663. https://doi.org/10.1177/13623613221122663. Online ahead of print	EXCLUDED—Article did not answer any research questions
35986472	Blair N	Comorbidities in Children with Autism Spectrum Disorder Undergoing Oral Rehabilitation Under General Anesthesia	*J Dent Child (Chic).* 2022 May 15;89(2):88–94	EXCLUDED—Article did not answer any research questions
35871424	Piraneh H	Social Story Based Toothbrushing Education Versus Video-Modeling Based Toothbrushing Training on Oral Hygiene Status Among Male Students Aged 7–15 Years Old with Autism Spectrum Disorders in Tehran, Iran: A Quasi-Randomized Controlled Trial	*J Autism Dev Disord.* 2022 Jul 24:1–12. https://doi.org/10.1007/s10803-022-05679-9. Online ahead of print	EXCLUDED—Article did not answer any research questions
35834048	Lilley R	"Peas in a pod": Oral History Reflections on Autistic Identity in Family and Community by Late-Diagnosed Adults	*J Autism Dev Disord.* 2022 Jul 14. https://doi.org/10.1007/s10803-022-05667-z. Online ahead of print	EXCLUDED—Article did not answer any research questions
35831693	Fenning RM	Optimizing Parent Training to Improve Oral Health Behavior and Outcomes in Underserved Children with Autism Spectrum Disorder	*J Autism Dev Disord.* 2022 Jul 14. https://doi.org/10.1007/s10803-022-05660-6. Online ahead of print	EXCLUDED—Article did not answer any research questions.

(continued)

(continued)

PubMed ID	First author	Article title	Citation information	Reason why the citation was either included or excluded
35626918	Floríndez LI	Toothbrushing and Oral Care Activities of Autistic and Non-Autistic Latino Children	*Children (Basel).* 2022 May 18;9(5):741. https://doi.org/10.3390/children9050741	EXCLUDED—Article did not answer any research questions
35455579	Carli E	Oral Health Preventive Program in Patients with Autism Spectrum Disorder	*Children (Basel).* 2022 Apr 10;9(4):535. https://doi.org/10.3390/children9040535	EXCLUDED—Article did not answer any research questions
35432796	Hajiahmadi M	Oral health knowledge, attitude, and performance of the parents of 3–12-year-old autistic children	*Dent Res J (Isfahan).* 2022 Mar 21;19:24. eCollection 2022	EXCLUDED—Article did not answer any research questions
35292925	Georgoula C	A Phase III Study of Bumetanide Oral Liquid Formulation for the Treatment of Children and Adolescents Aged Between 7 and 17 Years with Autism Spectrum Disorder (SIGN 1 Trial): Participant Baseline Characteristics	*Child Psychiatry Hum Dev.* 2022 Mar 16. https://doi.org/10.1007/s10578-022-01328-5. Online ahead of print	EXCLUDED—Article did not answer any research questions
35232533	Shalabi MASA	Picture Examination Communication System Versus Video Modelling in Improving Oral Hygiene of Children with Autism Spectrum Disorder: A Prospective Randomized Clinical Trial	*Pediatr Dent.* 2022 Jan 15;44(1):25–31	EXCLUDED—Article did not answer any research questions

(continued)

(continued)

PubMed ID	First author	Article title	Citation information	Reason why the citation was either included or excluded
35165451	Stewart Campbell A	Safety and target engagement of an oral small-molecule sequestrant in adolescents with autism spectrum disorder: an open-label phase 1b/2a trial	*Nat Med*. 2022 Mar;28(3):528–534. https://doi.org/10.1038/s41591-022-01683-9. Epub 2022 Feb 14	EXCLUDED—Article did not answer any research questions
35114831	Qiao Y	Oral Microbiota Changes Contribute to Autism Spectrum Disorder in Mice	*J Dent Res*. 2022 Jul;101(7):821–831. https://doi.org/10.1177/00220345211070470. Epub 2022 Feb 3	EXCLUDED—Study involved animals
35016051	Kaplan E	Intranasal dexmedetomidine vs oral triclofos sodium for sedation of children with autism undergoing electroencephalograms	*Eur J Paediatr Neurol*. 2022 Mar;37:19–24. https://doi.org/10.1016/j.ejpn.2022.01.005. Epub 2022 Jan 5	EXCLUDED—Article did not answer any research questions
34934690	Prakash J	Parental perception of oral health-related quality of life in children with autism. An observational study	*J Family Med Prim Care*. 2021 Oct;10(10):3845–3850. https://doi.org/10.4103/jfmpc.jfmpc_439_21. Epub 2021 Nov 5	EXCLUDED—Article did not answer any research questions
34925516	Bernath B	Exploring barriers to oral health care experienced by individuals living with autism spectrum disorder	*Can J Dent Hyg*. 2021 Oct 1;55(3):160–166. eCollection 2021 Oct	INCLUDED—This narrative literature review aims to raise awareness of the additional needs that individuals with ASD have when seeking oral care and to identify how barriers to such care may be reduced

(continued)

(continued)

PubMed ID	First author	Article title	Citation information	Reason why the citation was either included or excluded
34824512	Santosh A	Oral Health Assessment of Children with Autism Spectrum Disorder in Special Schools	*Int J Clin Pediatr Dent.* 2021 Jul–Aug;14(4):548–553. https://doi.org/10. 5005/jp-journals-10005-1972	EXCLUDED—Article did not answer any research questions
34760790	Chaware SH	The Systematic Review and Meta-analysis of Oral Sensory Challenges in Children and Adolescents with Autism Spectrum Disorder	*J Int Soc Prev Community Dent.* 2021 Aug 13;11(5):469–480. https://doi.org/10.4103/jis pcd.JISPCD_135_21. eCollection 2021 Sep–Oct	EXCLUDED—Article did not answer any research questions
34544255	Bagattoni S	Oral health status of Italian children with Autism Spectrum Disorder	*Eur J Paediatr Dent.* 2021 Sep;22(3):243–247. https://doi.org/10.23804/ ejpd.2021.22.03.12	EXCLUDED—Article did not answer any research questions
34440286	Mottron L	In Prototypical Autism, the Genetic Ability to Learn Language Is Triggered by Structured Information, Not Only by Exposure to Oral Language	*Genes (Basel).* 2021 Jul 22;12(8):1112. https:/ /doi.org/10.3390/genes12081112	EXCLUDED—Article did not answer any research questions
34376543	Mirsky LB	Oral Care Experiences of Young Adults with Autism Spectrum Disorder	*J Dent Hyg.* 2021 Aug;95(4):41–50	INCLUDED—The purpose of this study was to understand the oral healthcare experiences and needs of young adults with autism spectrum disorder

(continued)

(continued)

PubMed ID	First author	Article title	Citation information	Reason why the citation was either included or excluded
34335774	Fageeh HN	The Role of Applied Behavior Analysis to Improve Knowledge on Oral Hygiene Practices among Cooperative Autistic Children: A Cross-Sectional Study from Jazan, Saudi Arabia	*Int J Dent.* 2021 Jul 20:2021:9491496. https://doi.org/10.1155/2021/9491496. eCollection 2021	EXCLUDED—Article did not answer any research questions
34218395	Moorthy L	Dietary Sugar Exposure and Oral Health Status in Children with Autism Spectrum Disorder: A Case-control Study	*J Autism Dev Disord.* 2022 Jun;52(6):2523–2534. https://doi.org/10.1007/s10803-021-05151-0. Epub 2021 Jul 4	EXCLUDED—Article did not answer any research questions
34132672	Figueiredo T	The Recurrence of Motor Tics Mediated by Oral Prednisolone Use in Autistic Children: A Case Report	*Clin Neuropharmacol.* 2021 Ju–Aug 01:44(4):145–147. https://doi.org/10.1097/WNF.0000000000000463	EXCLUDED—Article did not answer any research questions
34050975	Krishnan L	Effectiveness of two sensory-based health education methods on oral hygiene of adolescent with autism spectrum disorders: An interventional study	*Spec Care Dentist.* 2021 Sep;41(5):626–633. https://doi.org/10.1111/scd.12606. Epub 2021 May 29	EXCLUDED—Article did not answer any research questions
33937604	Florindez LI	Identifying Gaps in Oral Care Knowledge, Attitudes, and Practices of Latinx Parents/Caregivers of Children With and Without Autism Spectrum Disorders	*Health Equity.* 2021 Apr 19;5(1):185–193. https://doi.org/10.1089/heq.2020.0078. eCollection 2021	EXCLUDED—Article did not answer any research questions

(continued)

PubMed ID	First author	Article title	Citation information	Reason why the citation was either included or excluded
33935841	DiCarlo GE	Autism-Associated Variant in the SLC6A3 Gene Alters the Oral Microbiome and Metabolism in a Murine Model	*Front Psychiatry*. 2021 Apr 15;12:655451. https://doi.org/10.3389/fpsyt.2021.655451. eCollection 2021	EXCLUDED—Article did not answer any research questions
33916808	Florindez LI	Exploring Eating Challenges and Food Selectivity for Latinx Children with and without Autism Spectrum Disorder Using Q ualitative Visual Methodology: Implications for Oral Health	*Int J Environ Res Public Health*. 2021 Apr 3;18(7):3751. https://doi.org/10.3390/ijerph 18073751	EXCLUDED—Article did not answer any research questions
33449432	Hammersmith KJ	Correlates of oral health fatalism in caregivers of children with autism spectrum disorder	*Spec Care Dentist*. 2021 Mar;41(2):145–153. https://doi.org/10.1111/scd.12564. Epub 2021 Jan 15	EXCLUDED—Article did not answer any research questions
33423216	Crutel V	Correction to: Bumetanide Oral Liquid Formulation for the Treatment of Children and Adolescents with Autism Spectrum Disorder: Design of Two Phase III Studies (SIGN Trials)	*J Autism Dev Disord*. 2021 Aug;51(8):2973. https://doi.org/10.1007/s10803-020-04822-8	EXCLUDED—This is a correction of a previous article
33375475	Como DH	Oral Health and Autism Spectrum Disorders: A Unique Collaboration between Dentistry and Occupational Therapy	*Int J Environ Res Public Health*. 2020 Dec 27;18(1):135. https://doi.org/10.3390/ijerph 18010135	EXCLUDED—Article did not answer any research questions
33257211	Kuter B	Evaluation of oral health status and oral disorders of children with autism spectrum disorders by gender	*Arch Pediatr*. 2021 Jan;28(1):33–38. https:// doi.org/10.1016/j.arcped.2020.10.009. Epub 2020 Nov 27	EXCLUDED—Article did not answer any research questions

(continued)

(continued)

(continued)

PubMed ID	First author	Article title	Citation information	Reason why the citation was either included or excluded
33151500	Crutel V	Bumetanide Oral Liquid Formulation for the Treatment of Children and Adolescents with Autism Spectrum Disorder: Design of Two Phase III Studies (SIGN Trials)	*J Autism Dev Disord.* 2021 Aug;51(8):2959–2972. https://doi.org/10.1007/s10803-020-04709-8	EXCLUDED—Article did not answer any research questions
33082718	AlHumaid J	Oral Health of Children with Autism: The Influence of Parental Attitudes and Willingness in Providing Care	*ScientificWorldJournal.* 2020 Oct 6;2020:8329426. https://doi.org/10.1155/2020/8329426. eCollection 2020	EXCLUDED—Article did not answer any research questions
32913567	Hage SRV	Oral hygiene and habits of children with autism spectrum disorders and their families	*J Clin Exp Dent.* 2020 Aug 1;12(8):e719–e724. https://doi.org/10.4317/jced.56440. eCollection 2020 Aug	EXCLUDED—Article did not answer any research questions
32812192	McBride GR	The Use of Oral Midazolam to Facilitate the Ophthalmic Examination of Children with Autism and Developmental Disorders	*J Autism Dev Disord.* 2021 May;51(5):1678–1682. https://doi.org/10.1007/s10803-020-04658-2	EXCLUDED—Article did not answer any research questions
32741583	Kosaka T	Low threshold to Vestibular and Oral Sensory stimuli might affect quality of sleep among children with autism spectrum disorder	*Brain Dev.* 2021 Jan;43(1):55–62. https://doi.org/10.1016/j.braindev.2020.07.010. Epub 2020 Jul 30	EXCLUDED—Article did not answer any research questions
32477184	Qiao Y	Oral Health Status of Chinese Children With Autism Spectrum Disorders	*Front Psychiatry.* 2020 May 5;11:398. https://doi.org/10.3389/fpsyt.2020.00398. eCollection 2020	EXCLUDED—Article did not answer any research questions
32474432	Pellicano E	Documenting the untold histories of late-diagnosed autistic adults: a qualitative study protocol using oral history methodology	*BMJ Open.* 2020 May 30;10(5):e037968. https://doi.org/10.1136/bmjopen-2020-037968	EXCLUDED—This study was a protocol

(continued)

(continued)

PubMed ID	First author	Article title	Citation information	Reason why the citation was either included or excluded
32323718	Corridore D	Prevalence of oral disease and treatment types proposed to children affected by Autistic Spectrum Disorder in Pediatric Dentistry: a Systematic Review	*Clin Ter.* 2020 May–Jun;171(3):e275–e282. https://doi.org/10.7417/CT.2020.2226	EXCLUDED—Article did not answer any research questions
32308277	Shah A	Caregiver's Sense of Coherence: A Predictor of Oral Health-Related Behaviors of Autistic Children in India	*Contemp Clin Dent.* 2019 Apr–Jun;10(2):197–202. https://doi.org/10. 4103/ccd.ccd_648_18	EXCLUDED—Article did not answer any research questions
32183521	Ferrazzano GF	Autism spectrum disorders and oral health status: review of the literature	*Eur J Paediatr Dent.* 2020 Mar;21(1):9–12. https://doi.org/10.23804/ejpd.2020.21.01.02	EXCLUDED—Article did not answer any research questions
32124144	Henry AR	Targeting Oral Language and Listening Comprehension Development for Students with Autism Spectrum Disorder: A School-Based Pilot Study	*J Autism Dev Disord.* 2020 Oct;50(10):3763–3776. https://doi.org/10. 1007/s10803-020-04434-2	EXCLUDED—Article did not answer any research questions
31995423	Pi X	A Meta-Analysis of Oral Health Status of Children with Autism	*J Clin Pediatr Dent.* 2020;44(1):1–7. https:// doi.org/10.17796/1053-4625-44.1.1	EXCLUDED—Article did not answer any research questions
31931609	Lam PP	Oral health status of children and adolescents with autism spectrum disorder: A systematic review of case–control studies and meta-analysis	*Autism.* 2020 Jul;24(5):1047–1066. https:// doi.org/10.1177/1362361319877337. Epub 2020 Jan 13	EXCLUDED—Article did not answer any research questions

(continued)

(continued)

PubMed ID	First author	Article title	Citation information	Reason why the citation was either included or excluded
31893019	Olsen I	Oral microbiota and autism spectrum disorder (ASD)	*J Oral Microbiol.* 2019 Dec 12;12(1):1702806. https://doi.org/10.1080/20002297.2019.1702806. eCollection 2020	EXCLUDED—Article did not answer any research questions
31802429	Du RY	Health- and oral health-related quality of life among preschool children with autism spectrum disorders	*Eur Arch Paediatr Dent.* 2020 Jun;21(3):363–371. https://doi.org/10.1007/s40368-019-00500-1. Epub 2019 Dec 4	EXCLUDED—Article did not answer any research questions
31787797	Zajic MC	Case studies comparing learning profiles and response to instruction in Autism Spectrum Disorder and Oral and Written Language Learning Disability at transition to high school	*Top Lang Disord.* 2019 Apr–Jun;39(2):128–154. https://doi.org/10.1097/TLD.0000000000000180	EXCLUDED—Article did not answer any research questions
31489949	Kong X	New and Preliminary Evidence on Altered Oral and Gut Microbiota in Individuals with Autism Spectrum Disorder (ASD): Implications for ASD Diagnosis and Subtyping Based on Microbial Biomarkers	*Nutrients.* 2019 Sep 6;11(9):2128. https://doi.org/10.3390/nu11092128	EXCLUDED—Article did not answer any research questions
31489825	Kuter B	Caries experience, oral disorders, oral hygiene practices and socio-demographic characteristics of autistic children	*Eur J Paediatr Dent.* 2019 Sep;20(3):237–241. https://doi.org/10.23804/ejpd.2019.20.03.13	EXCLUDED—Article did not answer any research questions
31489541	Leiva-García B	Association Between Feeding Problems and Oral Health Status in Children with Autism Spectrum Disorder	*J Autism Dev Disord.* 2019 Dec;49(12):4997–5008. https://doi.org/10.1007/s10803-019-04211-w	EXCLUDED—Article did not answer any research questions

(continued)

(continued)

PubMed ID	First author	Article title	Citation information	Reason why the citation was either included or excluded
31416123	Floríndez LI	Oral Care Experiences of Latino Parents/Caregivers with Children with Autism and with Typically Developing Children	*Int J Environ Res Public Health*. 2019 Aug 14;16(16):2905. https://doi.org/10.3390/ijerph16162905	EXCLUDED—Article did not answer any research questions
31339747	Wild H	Oral Contraceptives Reduced Pica Behavior in a Female with Autism Spectrum Disorder	*J Child Adolesc Psychopharmacol*. 2019 Dec;29(10):787. https://doi.org/10.1089/cap.2019.0094. Epub 2019 Jul 24	EXCLUDED—Article did not answer any research questions
31071244	Uezato A	Oral dysesthesia associated with autistic traits: a retrospective chart review	*Eur J Oral Sci*. 2019 Aug;127(4):347–350. https://doi.org/10.1111/eos.12620. Epub 2019 May 9	EXCLUDED—Article did not answer any research questions
31018497	Carrasco M	Alterations of Mitochondrial Biology in the Oral Mucosa of Chilean Children with Autism Spectrum Disorder (ASD)	*Cells*. 2019 Apr 23:8(4):367. https://doi.org/10.3390/cells8040367	EXCLUDED—Article did not answer any research questions
30803480	Stein Duker LI	Strategies for Success: A Qualitative Study of Caregiver and Dentist Approaches to Improving Oral Care for Children with Autism	*Pediatr Dent*. 2019 Jan 15:41(1):4E–12E	INCLUDED—The purpose of this study was to qualitatively explore parental and dentist reports of successful strategies implemented during dental care with autistic children
30687090	Barchel D	Oral Cannabidiol Use in Children With Autism Spectrum Disorder to Treat Related Symptoms and Co-morbidities	*Front Pharmacol*. 2019 Jan 9;9:1521. https://doi.org/10.3389/fphar.2018.01521. eCollection 2018	EXCLUDED—Article did not answer any research questions

(continued)

(continued)

PubMed ID	First author	Article title	Citation information	Reason why the citation was either included or excluded
30681777	Wang X	Oral probiotic administration during pregnancy prevents autism-related behaviors in offspring induced by maternal immune activation via anti-inflammation in mice	*Autism Res.* 2019 Apr;12(4):576–588. https://doi.org/10.1002/aur.2079. Epub 2019 Jan 25	EXCLUDED—Article did not answer any research questions
30573708	Orellana LM	Psychoeducational intervention to improve oral assessment in people with autism spectrum disorder, BIO-BIO region, Chile	*Med Oral Patol Oral Cir Bucal.* 2019 Jan 1;24(1):e37-e46. https://doi.org/10.4317/medoral.22560	EXCLUDED—Article did not answer any research questions
30542908	Lefer G	Training children with autism spectrum disorder to undergo oral assessment using a digital iPad® application	*Eur Arch Paediatr Dent.* 2019 Apr;20(2):113–121. https://doi.org/10.1007/s40368-018-0398-9. Epub 2018 Dec 12	INCLUDED—To present a training programme for teaching autistic children and adolescents to be compliant with a dental examination *THIS STUDY COULD NOT BE ACCESSED*
30314501	Naidoo M	The Oral health status of children with autism Spectrum disorder in KwaZulu-Nata, South Africa	*BMC Oral Health.* 2018 Oct 12;18(1):165. https://doi.org/10.1186/s12903-018-0632-1	EXCLUDED—Article did not answer any research questions
30178105	Vargason T	Gastrointestinal Symptoms and Oral Antibiotic Use in Children with Autism Spectrum Disorder: Retrospective Analysis of a Privately Insured U.S. Population	*J Autism Dev Disord.* 2019 Feb;49(2):647–659. https://doi.org/10.1007/s10803-018-3743-2	EXCLUDED—Article did not answer any research questions

(continued)

(continued)

PubMed ID	First author	Article title	Citation information	Reason why the citation was either included or excluded
30107083	Hicks SD	Oral microbiome activity in children with autism spectrum disorder	*Autism Res.* 2018 Sep;11(9):1286–1299. https://doi.org/10.1002/aur.1972. Epub 2018 Aug 14	EXCLUDED—Article did not answer any research questions
30085870	Eslami N	Parents' Perceptions of the Oral Health-related Quality of Life of their Autistic Children in Iran	*J Clin Pediatr Dent.* 2018;42(6):422–426. https://doi.org/10.17796/1053-4625-42.6.3. Epub 2018 Aug 7	EXCLUDED—Article did not answer any research questions
29983812	Kotha SB	Associations between Diet, Dietary and Oral Hygiene Habits with Caries Occurrence and Severity in Children with Autism at Dammam City, Saudi Arabia	*Open Access Maced J Med Sci.* 2018 Jun 6;6(6):1104–1110. https://doi.org/10.3889/oamjms.2018.245. eCollection 2018 Jun 20	EXCLUDED—Article did not answer any research questions
33073267	Parish-Morris J	Oral-Motor and Lexical Diversity During Naturalistic Conversations in Adults with Autism Spectrum Disorder	*Proc Conf.* 2018 Jun;2018:147–157. https://doi.org/10.18653/v1/w18-0616	EXCLUDED—Article did not answer any research questions
29790776	Mansoor D	Oral health challenges facing Dubai children with Autism Spectrum Disorder at home and in accessing oral health care	*Eur J Paediatr Dent.* 2018 Jun;19(2):127–133. https://doi.org/10.23804/ejpd.2018.19.02.06	INCLUDED—To investigate the challenges faced by autistic children and their families in Dubai from three different perspectives of dental care: oral care at home, oral care at the dentist and access to oral care, and to compare the results to their normally developing peers

(continued)

(continued)

PubMed ID	First author	Article title	Citation information	Reason why the citation was either included or excluded
29607853	Onol S	Evaluation of oral health status and influential factors in children with autism	*Niger J Clin Pract*. 2018 Apr;21(4):429–435. https://doi.org/10.4103/njcp.njcp_41_17	EXCLUDED—Article did not answer any research questions
29575458	Stuker EW	Third time's a charm: Oral midazolam vs intranasal dexmedetomidine for preoperative anxiolysis in an autistic pediatric patient	*Paediatr Anaesth*. 2018 Apr;28(4):370–371. https://doi.org/10.1111/pan.13335	EXCLUDED—Article did not answer any research questions
29460795	Good P	Evidence the U.S. autism epidemic initiated by acetaminophen (Tylenol) is aggravated by oral antibiotic amoxicillin/clavulanate (Augmentin) and now exponentially by herbicide glyphosate (Roundup)	*Clin Nutr ESPEN*. 2018 Feb;23:171–183. https://doi.org/10.1016/j.clnesp.2017.10.005. Epub 2017 Dec 1	EXCLUDED—Article did not answer any research questions
29371629	Qiao Y	Alterations of oral microbiota distinguish children with autism spectrum disorders from healthy controls	*Sci Rep*. 2018 Jan 25;8(1):1597. https://doi.org/10.1038/s41598-018-19982-y	EXCLUDED—Article did not answer any research questions
29269185	Rouches A	Tools and techniques to improve the oral health of children with autism	*Arch Pediatr*. 2018 Feb;25(2):145–149. https://doi.org/10.1016/j.arcped.2017.11.013	EXCLUDED—This article is published in French
29076744	Suhaib F	Oral assessment of children with autism spectrum disorder in Rawalpindi, Pakistan	*Autism*. 2019 Jan;23(1):81–86. https://doi.org/10.1177/1362361317730299. Epub 2017 Oct 27	EXCLUDED—Article did not answer any research questions

(continued)

(continued)

PubMed ID	First author	Article title	Citation information	Reason why the citation was either included or excluded
36249785	Stolar O	Medical cannabis for the treatment of comorbid symptoms in children with autism spectrum disorder: An interim analysis of biochemical safety	*Front Pharmacol.* 2022 Sep 29;13:977484. https://doi.org/10.3389/fphar.2022.977484. eCollection 2022	EXCLUDED—Article did not answer any research questions
36159065	Erridge S	Clinical outcome analysis of patients with autism spectrum disorder: analysis from the UK Medical Cannabis Registry	*Ther Adv Psychopharmacol.* 2022 Sep 20;12:20451253221116240. https://doi.org/10.1177/20451253221116240. eCollection 2022	EXCLUDED—Article did not answer any research questions
36053627	Dhuga Y	Developing undergraduate autism education for medical students: a qualitative study	*BMJ Paediatr Open.* 2022 Aug;6(1):e001411. https://doi.org/10.1136/bmjpo-2022-001411	EXCLUDED—Article did not answer any research questions
35820787	Alberts LB	Preliminary Development and Testing of the Risk Assessment Checklist for Self-Injury in Autism-Medical (RACSA-M)	*J Dr Nurs Pract.* 2022 Jul 1;15(2):75–83. https://doi.org/10.1891/JDNP-2021-0034	EXCLUDED—Article did not answer any research questions
35766927	ANONYMOUS	Medical Management of Children With Autism in the Emergency Department	*Pediatr Emerg Care.* 2022 Jul 1;38(7):337–338. https://doi.org/10.1097/01. pec.0000852776.33130.0c	EXCLUDED—Article did not answer any research questions
35766926	ANONYMOUS	Medical Management of Children With Autism in the Emergency Department	*Pediatr Emerg Care.* 2022 Jul 1;38(7):462–463. https://doi.org/10.1097/ PEC.0000000000002751	EXCLUDED—Article did not answer any research questions
35653008	Ezeh TH	The Medical Home and Use of Mental and Non-mental Specialty Services Among Children with Autism Spectrum Disorder (ASD)	*J Autism Dev Disord.* 2022 Jun 2. https://doi. org/10.1007/s10803-022-05596-x. Online ahead of print	EXCLUDED—Article did not answer any research questions

(continued)

(continued)

PubMed ID	First author	Article title	Citation information	Reason why the citation was either included or excluded
35513550	Megerian JT	Evaluation of an artificial intelligence-based medical device for diagnosis of autism spectrum disorder	*NPJ Digit Med.* 2022 May 5;5(1):57. https://doi.org/10.1038/s41746-022-00598-6	EXCLUDED—Article did not answer any research questions
35343818	Siani-Rose M	The Potential of Salivary Lipid-Based Cannabis-Responsive Biomarkers to Evaluate Medical Cannabis Treatment in Children with Autism Spectrum Disorder	*Cannabis Cannabinoid Res.* 2022 Mar 28. https://doi.org/10.1089/can.2021.0224. Online ahead of print	EXCLUDED—Article did not answer any research questions
35338618	Ashikin MN	The prevalence of Autism Spectrum Disorder in Down Syndrome children attending the Child Development Centre in Universiti Kebangsaan Malaysia Medical Centre	*Med J Malaysia.* 2022 Mar;77(2):137–142	EXCLUDED—Article did not answer any research questions
35305752	Shaw SCK	Challenging the exclusion of autistic medical students	*Lancet Psychiatry.* 2022 Apr;9(4):e18. https://doi.org/10.1016/S2215-0366(22)00061-X	EXCLUDED—Article did not answer any research questions
35284942	Badgett NM	Emergency Department Utilization Among Youth with Autism Spectrum Disorder: Exploring the Role of Preventive Care, Medical Home, and Mental Health Access	*J Autism Dev Disord.* 2022 Mar 14. https://doi.org/10.1007/s10803-022-05503-4. Online ahead of print	EXCLUDED—Article did not answer any research questions
35194015	Carlsson T	Association of cumulative early medical factors with autism and autistic symptoms in a population-based twin sample	*Transl Psychiatry.* 2022 Feb 22;12(1):73. https://doi.org/10.1038/s41398-022-01833-0	EXCLUDED—Article did not answer any research questions

(continued)

(continued)

PubMed ID	First author	Article title	Citation information	Reason why the citation was either included or excluded
35012536	Mukhamedshina YO	Health care providers' awareness on medical management of children with autism spectrum disorder: cross-sectional study in Russia	*BMC Med Educ.* 2022 Jan 10;22(1):29. https://doi.org/10.1186/s12909-021-03095-8	EXCLUDED—Article did not answer any research questions
34948647	Al-Mazidi SH	National Profile of Caregivers' Perspectives on Autism Spectrum Disorder Screening and Care in Primary Health Care: The Need for Autism Medical Home	*Int J Environ Res Public Health.* 2021 Dec 10;18(24):13043. https://doi.org/10.3390/ijerph182413043	EXCLUDED—Article did not answer any research questions
34874191	Siani-Rose M	Cannabis-Responsive Biomarkers: A Pharmacometabolomics-Based Application to Evaluate the Impact of Medical Cannabis Treatment on Children with Autism Spectrum Disorder	*Cannabis Cannabinoid Res.* 2021 Dec 6. https://doi.org/10.1089/can.2021.0129. Online ahead of print	EXCLUDED—Article did not answer any research questions
34859733	Shaw SCK	Autistic role modelling in medical education	*Educ Prim Care.* 2022 Mar;33(2):128–129. https://doi.org/10.1080/14739879.2021.1996277. Epub 2021 Dec 3	EXCLUDED—Article did not answer any research questions
34853956	Eyoh EE	Brief Report: The Characterization of Medical Comorbidity Prior to Autism Diagnosis in Children Before Age Two	*J Autism Dev Disord.* 2021 Dec 1:10.1007/s10803-021-05380-3. https://doi.org/10.1007/s10803-021-05380-3. Online ahead of print	EXCLUDED—Article did not answer any research questions

(continued)

(continued)

PubMed ID	First author	Article title	Citation information	Reason why the citation was either included or excluded
34737666	Watanabe T	Association of Autism Spectrum Disorder and Attention Deficit Hyperactivity Disorder Traits with Depression and Empathy Among Medical Students	*Adv Med Educ Pract*. 2021 Oct 28;12:1259–1265. https://doi.org/10.2147/AMEP.S334155. eCollection 2021	EXCLUDED—Article did not answer any research questions
34683092	Grivas G	Pregnant Mothers' Medical Claims and Associated Risk of Their Children being Diagnosed with Autism Spectrum Disorder	*J Pers Med*. 2021 Sep 24;11(10):950. https://doi.org/10.3390/jpm11100950	EXCLUDED—Article did not answer any research questions
34645786	Poleg S	Behavioral aspects and neurobiological properties underlying medical cannabis treatment in Shank3 mouse model of autism spectrum disorder	*Transl Psychiatry*. 2021 Oct 13;11(1):524. https://doi.org/10.1038/s41398-021-01612-3	EXCLUDED—Study involved animals
34432543	Holdman R	Safety and Efficacy of Medical Cannabis in Autism Spectrum Disorder Compared with Commonly Used Medications	*Cannabis Cannabinoid Res*. 2022 Aug;7(4):451–463. https://doi.org/10.1089/can.2020.0154. Epub 2021 Aug 24	EXCLUDED—Article did not answer any research questions
34376162	Shawahna R	Are medical students in Palestine adequately trained to care for individuals with autism spectrum disorders? A multicenter cross-sectional study of their familiarity, knowledge, confidence, and willingness to learn	*BMC Med Educ*. 2021 Aug 10;21(1):424. https://doi.org/10.1186/s12909-021-02865-8	INCLUDED—The present study was undertaken to assess familiarity, knowledge, confidence, of medical students about autism spectrum disorders (ASDs)

(continued)

(continued)

PubMed ID	First author	Article title	Citation information	Reason why the citation was either included or excluded
34184558	Simantov T	Medical symptoms and conditions in autistic women	*Autism.* 2022 Feb;26(2):373–388. https://doi.org/10.1177/13623613211022091. Epub 2021 Jun 29	EXCLUDED—Article did not answer any research questions
34146208	Strang JF	Transgender Youth Executive Functioning: Relationships with Anxiety Symptoms, Autism Spectrum Disorder, and Gender-Affirming Medical Treatment Status	*Child Psychiatry Hum Dev.* 2022 Dec;53(6):1252–1265. https://doi.org/10.1007/s10578-021-01195-6. Epub 2021 Jun 19	EXCLUDED—Article did not answer any research questions
33972922	Al-Beltagi M	Autism medical comorbidities	*World J Clin Pediatr.* 2021 May 9;10(3):15–28. https://doi.org/10.5409/wjcp.v10.i3.15. eCollection 2021 May 9	EXCLUDED—This was an editorial
36324994	Ejlskov L	Prediction of Autism Risk From Family Medical History Data Using Machine Learning: A National Cohort Study From Denmark	*Biol Psychiatry Glob Open Sci.* 2021 May 5;1(2):156–164. https://doi.org/10.1016/j.bpsgos.2021.04.007. eCollection 2021 Aug	EXCLUDED—Article did not answer any research questions
33936398	Brown KA	Mental Health Comorbidity Analysis in Pediatric Patients with Autism Spectrum Disorder Using Rhode Island Medical Claims Data	*AMIA Annu Symp Proc.* 2021 Jan 25;2020:263–272. eCollection 2020	EXCLUDED—Article did not answer any research questions
33914226	Rast J	Health Service and Functional Measures of Benefit of a Medical Home in Children with Autism	*Matern Child Health J.* 2021 Jul;25(7):1156–1163. https://doi.org/10.1007/s10995-021-03150-2. Epub 2021 Apr 29	EXCLUDED—Article did not answer any research questions
33611772	Giroux M	Shedding light on autistic traits in struggling learners: A blind spot in medical education	*Perspect Med Educ.* 2021 Jun;10(3):180–186. https://doi.org/10.1007/s40037-021-00654-z. Epub 2021 Feb 20	EXCLUDED—Article did not answer any research questions

(continued)

(continued)

PubMed ID	First author	Article title	Citation information	Reason why the citation was either included or excluded
33526241	Wisner-Carlson RW	Acts of Medical Kindness for People with Autism	*Psychiatr Clin North Am.* 2021 Mar;44(1):xi–xiv. https://doi.org/10.1016/j.psc.2021.01.001	EXCLUDED—This was an editorial
33271720	Goh TJ	Supporting individuals with Autism Spectrum Disorder in medical settings during COVID-19	*Asian J Psychiatr.* 2020 Dec;54:102441. https://doi.org/10.1016/j.ajp.2020.102441. Epub 2020 Oct 9	EXCLUDED—This was an editorial
33238726	Harris JF	Development and implementation of health care transition resources for youth with autism spectrum disorders within a primary care medical home	*Autism.* 2021 Apr;25(3):753–766. https://doi.org/10.1177/1362361320974491. Epub 2020 Nov 25	EXCLUDED—Article did not answer any research questions
33098262	Brooks JD	Identifying Children and Youth With Autism Spectrum Disorder in Electronic Medical Records: Examining Health System Utilization and Comorbidities	*Autism Res.* 2021 Feb;14(2):400–410. https://doi.org/10.1002/aur.2419. Epub 2020 Oct 24	EXCLUDED—Article did not answer any research questions
33082092	Snyder J	Crowdfunding, stem cell interventions and autism spectrum disorder: comparing campaigns related to an international "stem cell clinic" and US academic medical center	*Cytotherapy.* 2021 Mar;23(3):198–202. https://doi.org/10.1016/j.jcyt.2020.09.002. Epub 2020 Oct 17	EXCLUDED—Article did not answer any research questions
33068218	Kouo JL	A Scoping Review of Targeted Interventions and Training to Facilitate Medical Encounters for School-Aged Patients with an Autism Spectrum Disorder	*J Autism Dev Disord.* 2021 Aug;51(8):2829–2851. https://doi.org/10.1007/s10803-020-04716-9	EXCLUDED—Article did not answer any research questions

(continued)

(continued)

PubMed ID	First author	Article title	Citation information	Reason why the citation was either included or excluded
32972657	Ferrari E	Dealing with confounders and outliers in classification medical studies: The Autism Spectrum Disorders case study	*Artif Intell Med.* 2020 Aug;108:101926. https://doi.org/10.1016/j.artmed.2020.101926. Epub 2020 Jul 6	EXCLUDED—Article did not answer any research questions
32960953	Anderson MP	Autism BrainNet: A Collaboration Between Medical Examiners, Pathologists, Researchers, and Families to Advance the Understanding and Treatment of Autism Spectrum Disorder	*Arch Pathol Lab Med.* 2021 Apr 1;145(4):494–501. https://doi.org/10.5858/arpa.2020-0164-RA	EXCLUDED—Article did not answer any research questions
32907353	Hand BN	Specialized primary care medical home: A positive impact on continuity of care among autistic adults	*Autism.* 2021 Jan;25(1):258–265. https://doi.org/10.1177/1362361320953967. Epub 2020 Sep 9	EXCLUDED—Article did not answer any research questions
32907348	Gilmore D	Health status of Medicare-enrolled autistic older adults with and without co-occurring intellectual disability: An analysis of inpatient and institutional outpatient medical claims	*Autism.* 2021 Jan;25(1):266–274. https://doi.org/10.1177/1362361320955109. Epub 2020 Sep 9	EXCLUDED—Article did not answer any research questions
32900813	Thom RP	Providing Inpatient Medical Care to Children With Autism Spectrum Disorder	*Hosp Pediatr.* 2020 Oct;10(10):918–924. https://doi.org/10.1542/hpeds.2020-0140. Epub 2020 Sep 8	EXCLUDED—Article did not answer any research questions
32892960	Mostafavi M	Autism Spectrum Disorder and Medical Cannabis: Review and Clinical Experience	*Semin Pediatr Neurol.* 2020 Oct;35:100833. https://doi.org/10.1016/j.spen.2020.100833. Epub 2020 Jul 2	EXCLUDED—Article did not answer any research questions

(continued)

(continued)

PubMed ID	First author	Article title	Citation information	Reason why the citation was either included or excluded
32662293	Failla MD	Using phecode analysis to characterize co-occurring medical conditions in autism spectrum disorder	*Autism.* 2021 Apr;25(3):800–811. https://doi.org/10.1177/1362361320934561. Epub 2020 Jul 14	EXCLUDED—Article did not answer any research questions
32560589	Limbers CA	The Patient-Centered Medical Home: Mental Health and Parenting Stress in Mothers of Children With Autism	*J Prim Care Community Health.* 2020 Jan–Dec;11:2150132720936067. https://doi.org/10.1177/2150132720936067	EXCLUDED—Article did not answer any research questions
32494255	Akhter N	Autism Cognizance: A dilemma among medical and Allied Medical practitioners	*Pak J Med Sci.* 2020 May–Jun;36(4):678–682. https://doi.org/10.12669/pjms.36.4.1703	EXCLUDED—Article did not answer any research questions
32471603	Wisner-Carlson RW	Acts of Medical Kindness for People with Autism	*Child Adolesc Psychiatr Clin N Am.* 2020 Jul;29(3):xi–xiv. https://doi.org/10.1016/j.chc.2020.03.005. Epub 2020 Apr 23	EXCLUDED—This was an editorial
32389225	Leibson C	Objective Estimates of Direct-Medical Costs Among Persons Aged 3 to 38 Years With and Without Research-Defined Autism Spectrum Disorder Ascertained During Childhood: A Population-Based Birth-Cohort Study	*Value Health.* 2020 May;23(5):595–605. https://doi.org/10.1016/j.jval.2019.12.006. Epub 2020 Feb 27	EXCLUDED—Article did not answer any research questions
32341146	Oztan O	Neonatal CSF vasopressin concentration predicts later medical record diagnoses of autism spectrum disorder	*Proc Natl Acad Sci U S A.* 2020 May 12;117(19):10609–10613. https://doi.org/10.1073/pnas.1919050117. Epub 2020 Apr 27	EXCLUDED—Article did not answer any research questions

(continued)

(continued)

PubMed ID	First author	Article title	Citation information	Reason why the citation was either included or excluded
32319096	Dufour MM	Increasing compliance with wearing a medical device in children with autism	*J Appl Behav Anal*. 2020 Apr;53(2):1089–1096. https://doi.org/10.1002/jaba.628. Epub 2019 Sep 2	EXCLUDED—Article did not answer any research questions
32238537	Hazen EP	Agitation in Patients With Autism Spectrum Disorder Admitted to Inpatient Pediatric Medical Units	*Pediatrics*. 2020 Apr;145(Suppl 1):S108–S116. https://doi.org/10.1542/peds.2019-1895N	EXCLUDED—Article did not answer any research questions
32140022	Patra S	Symptom Recognition to Diagnosis: Pathway to Care for Autism in a Tertiary Care Medical Centre	*J Neurosci Rural Pract*. 2020 Jan;11(1):164–169. https://doi.org/10.1055/s-0040-1701778. Epub 2020 Mar 3	EXCLUDED—Article did not answer any research questions
32125565	Cohen IL	Triggers of Aggressive Behaviors in Intellectually Disabled Adults and Their Association with Autism, Medical Conditions, Psychiatric Disorders, Age and Sex: A Large-Scale Study	*J Autism Dev Disord*. 2020 Oct;50(10):3748–3762. https://doi.org/10.1007/s10803-020-04424-4	EXCLUDED—Article did not answer any research questions
32100657	Rahman R	Identification of newborns at risk for autism using electronic medical records and machine learning	*Eur Psychiatry*. 2020 Feb 26;63(1):e22. https://doi.org/10.1192/j.eurpsy.2020.17	EXCLUDED—Article did not answer any research questions
32096123	Fombonne E	Psychiatric and Medical Profiles of Autistic Adults in the SPARK Cohort	*J Autism Dev Disord*. 2020 Oct;50(10):3679–3698. https://doi.org/10.1007/s10803-020-04414-6	EXCLUDED—Article did not answer any research questions

(continued)

(continued)

PubMed ID	First author	Article title	Citation information	Reason why the citation was either included or excluded
31583622	Jensen EJ	Working with Children with Autism Spectrum Disorder in a Medical Setting: Insights from Certified Child Life Specialists	*J Autism Dev Disord.* 2020 Jan;50(1):189–198. https://doi.org/10.1007/s10803-019-04245-0	EXCLUDED—This study aimed to gain an understanding of Certified Child Life Specialists' experiences with and suggestions for working with autistic children in a medical setting This study was later excluded since it did not answer any research questions
31473462	Koren G	Corrigendum to: "Does high-dose gestational folic acid increase the risk for autism? The birth order hypothesis" [Medical Hypotheses 132 (2019) 109350]	*Med Hypotheses.* 2019 Dec;133:109378. https://doi.org/10.1016/j.mehy.2019.109378. Epub 2019 Aug 29	EXCLUDED—This was a published erratum
31422989	Jones KB	Cost and Utilization with Enrollment in a Medical Home for Individuals with an Autism Spectrum Disorder and/or Intellectual Disability	*J Health Care Poor Underserved.* 2019;30(3):1068–1082. https://doi.org/10.1353/hpu.2019.0074	EXCLUDED—Article did not answer any research questions
31415008	Hawkins JR	Bergamot Aromatherapy for Medical Office-Induced Anxiety Among Children With an Autism Spectrum Disorder: A Randomized, Controlled, Blinded Clinical Trial	*Holist Nurs Pract.* 2019 Sep/Oct;33(5):285–294. https://doi.org/10.1097/HNP.0000000000000341	EXCLUDED—Article did not answer any research questions

(continued)

(continued)

PubMed ID	First author	Article title	Citation information	Reason why the citation was either included or excluded
31316404	Tye C	Corrigendum: Characterizing the Interplay Between Autism Spectrum Disorder and Comorbid Medical Conditions: An Integrative Review	*Front Psychiatry*. 2019 Jun 27;10:438. https://doi.org/10.3389/fpsyt.2019.00438. eCollection 2019	EXCLUDED—This was a published erratum
31243575	Shefer S	Benefits of medical clowning in the treatment of young children with autism spectrum disorder	*Eur J Pediatr*. 2019 Aug;178(8):1283–1289. https://doi.org/10.1007/s00431-019-03415-7. Epub 2019 Jun 26	EXCLUDED—Article did not answer any research questions
31174865	Thom RP	Challenges in the Medical Care of Patients With Autism Spectrum Disorder: The Role of the Consultation-Liaison Psychiatrist	*Psychosomatics*. 2019 Sep–Oct;60(5):435–443. https://doi.org/10.1016/j.psym.2019.04.003. Epub 2019 Apr 28	EXCLUDED—Article did not answer any research questions
31164130	Li HJ	Utilization and medical costs of outpatient rehabilitation among children with autism spectrum conditions in Taiwan	*BMC Health Serv Res*. 2019 Jun 4;19(1):354. https://doi.org/10.1186/s12913-019-4193-z	EXCLUDED—Article did not answer any research questions
31149786	Vargason T	Clustering of co-occurring conditions in autism spectrum disorder during early childhood: A retrospective analysis of medical claims data	*Autism Res*. 2019 Aug;12(8):1272–1285. https://doi.org/10.1002/aur.2128. Epub 2019 May 31	EXCLUDED—Article did not answer any research questions
31144278	Brondino N	Prevalence of Medical Comorbidities in Adults with Autism Spectrum Disorder	*J Gen Intern Med*. 2019 Oct;34(10):1992–1994. https://doi.org/10.1007/s11606-019-05071-x	EXCLUDED—Article did not answer any research questions

(continued)

(continued)

PubMed ID	First author	Article title	Citation information	Reason why the citation was either included or excluded
31065222	Straus J	Medical Encounters for Youth With Autism Spectrum Disorder: A Comprehensive Review of Environmental Considerations and Interventions	*Clin Med Insights Pediatr.* 2019 Apr 29;13:1179556519842816. https://doi.org/10.1177/1179556519842816. eCollection 2019	EXCLUDED—Article did not answer any research questions
31007427	Ellias SD	A Study of Assessment of Knowledge of Childhood Autism among Medical Students in Mumbai	*Ann Indian Acad Neurol.* 2019 Apr–Jun;22(2):164–169. https://doi.org/10.4103/aian.AIAN_486_17	EXCLUDED—Article did not answer any research questions
30947543	Mello S	Physician Mediation Theory and Pediatric Media Guidance in the Digital Age: A Survey of Autism Medical and Clinical Professionals	*Health Commun.* 2020 Jul;35(8):955–965. https://doi.org/10.1080/10410236.2019.1598744. Epub 2019 Apr 5	EXCLUDED—Article did not answer any research questions
30838668	Turowetz J	Documenting diagnosis: testing, labelling, and the production of medical records in an autism clinic	*Sociol Health Illn.* 2019 Jul;41(6):1023–1039. https://doi.org/10.1111/1467-9566.12882. Epub 2019 Mar 5	EXCLUDED—Article did not answer any research questions
30820126	Trüeb RM	Autistic-Undisciplined Thinking in the Practice of Medical Trichology	*Int J Trichology.* 2019 Jan–Feb;11(1):1–7. https://doi.org/10.4103/ijt.ijt_79_18	EXCLUDED—Article did not answer any research questions
30733689	Tye C	Characterizing the Interplay Between Autism Spectrum Disorder and Comorbid Medical Conditions: An Integrative Review	*Front Psychiatry.* 2019 Jan 23;9:751. https://doi.org/10.3389/fpsyt.2018.00751. eCollection 2018	EXCLUDED—Article did not answer any research questions
30655581	Bar-Lev Schleider L	Real life Experience of Medical Cannabis Treatment in Autism: Analysis of Safety and Efficacy	*Sci Rep.* 2019 Jan 17;9(1):200. https://doi.org/10.1038/s41598-018-37570-y	EXCLUDED—Article did not answer any research questions

(continued)

(continued)

PubMed ID	First author	Article title	Citation information	Reason why the citation was either included or excluded
30352916	Hayes AL	Autism Spectrum Disorder: Patient Care Strategies for Medical Imaging	*Radiol Technol.* 2018 Sep;90(1):31–47	EXCLUDED—Article did not answer any research questions
30136407	Wilson SA	Medical care experiences of children with autism and their parents: A scoping review	*Child Care Health Dev.* 2018 Nov;44(6):807–817. https://doi.org/10.1111/cch.12611. Epub 2018 Aug 22	INCLUDED—This review examined literature that describes experiences in medical care settings from the perspective of patients under age 18 with ASD and their caregivers
30053632	Neumeyer AM	Identifying Associations Among Co-Occurring Medical Conditions in Children With Autism Spectrum Disorders	*Acad Pediatr.* 2019 Apr;19(3):300–306. https://doi.org/10.1016/j.acap.2018.06.014. Epub 2018 Jul 24	EXCLUDED—Article did not answer any research questions
30005820	Sharp WG	Dietary Intake, Nutrient Status, and Growth Parameters in Children with Autism Spectrum Disorder and Severe Food Selectivity: An Electronic Medical Record Review	*J Acad Nutr Diet.* 2018 Oct;118(10):1943–1950. https://doi.org/10.1016/j.jand.2018.05.005. Epub 2018 Jul 10	EXCLUDED—Article did not answer any research questions
29719986	Shahidullah JD	Linking the Medical and Educational Home to Support Children With Autism Spectrum Disorder: Practice Recommendations	*Clin Pediatr (Phila).* 2018 Nov;57(13):1496–1505. https://doi.org/10.1177/0009922818774344. Epub 2018 May 3	EXCLUDED—Article did not answer any research questions
29610414	Rast JE	The Medical Home and Health Care Transition for Youth With Autism	*Pediatrics.* 2018 Apr;141(Suppl 4):S328–S334. https://doi.org/10.1542/peds.2016-4300J	EXCLUDED—Article did not answer any research questions

(continued)

PubMed ID	First author	Article title	Citation information	Reason why the citation was either included or excluded
29589272	Hine JF	Embedding Autism Spectrum Disorder Diagnosis Within the Medical Home: Decreasing Wait Times Through Streamlined Assessment	*J Autism Dev Disord.* 2018 Aug;48(8):2846–2853. https://doi.org/10.1007/s10803-018-3548-3	EXCLUDED—Article did not answer any research questions
29524016	Soke GN	Prevalence of Co-occurring Medical and Behavioral Conditions/Symptoms Among 4- and 8-Year-Old Children with Autism Spectrum Disorder in Selected Areas of the United States in 2010	*J Autism Dev Disord.* 2018 Aug;48(8):2663–2676. https://doi.org/10.1007/s10803-018-3521-1	EXCLUDED—Article did not answer any research questions
29389684	Todorow C	The medical home for children with autism spectrum disorder: an essential element whose time has come	*Curr Opin Pediatr.* 2018 Apr;30(2):311–317. https://doi.org/10.1097/MOP.0000000000000605	EXCLUDED—Article did not answer any research questions
29298245	Cheung V	Emergency Medical Responders and Adolescents With Autism Spectrum Disorder	*Pediatr Emerg Care.* 2019 Apr;35(4):273–277. https://doi.org/10.1097/PEC.0000000000001322	EXCLUDED—Article did not answer any research questions
28750547	Saqr Y	Addressing medical needs of adolescents and adults with autism spectrum disorders in a primary care setting	*Autism.* 2018 Jan;22(1):51–61. https://doi.org/10.1177/1362361317709970. Epub 2017 Jul 28	EXCLUDED—Article did not answer any research questions
28203249	Yuan J	Autism spectrum disorder detection from semi-structured and unstructured medical data	*EURASIP J Bioinform Syst Biol.* 2017 Feb 1;2017:3. https://doi.org/10.1186/s13637-017-0057-1. eCollection 2017 Dec	EXCLUDED—Article did not answer any research questions

(continued)

(continued)

PubMed ID	First author	Article title	Citation information	Reason why the citation was either included or excluded
36358360	Samadi SA	The Challenges of Establishing Healthcare Services in Low- and Middle-Income Countries: The Case of Autism Spectrum Disorders (ASD) in the Kurdistan Region of Iraq-Report from the Field	*Brain Sci.* 2022 Oct 25;12(11):1433. https://doi.org/10.3390/brainsci12111433	EXCLUDED—Article did not answer any research questions
36189783	Underwood JFG	Neurological and psychiatric disorders among autistic adults: a population healthcare record study	*Psychol Med.* 2022 Oct 3:1–11. https://doi.org/10.1017/S0033291722002884. Online ahead of print	EXCLUDED—Article did not answer any research questions
36149418	Kyle G	Developing an e-learning curriculum to educate healthcare staff in the acute hospital setting about autism	*Br J Nurs.* 2022 Sep 22;31(17):894–900. https://doi.org/10.12968/bjon.2022.31.17.894	EXCLUDED—Article did not answer any research questions
36043964	Conte L	Autism Spectrum Disorders and inclusion attitudes in the Italian school environments: teachers' knowledge, attitudes, perceptions and their necessity to consult a healthcare multidisciplinary team	*Acta Biomed.* 2022 Aug 31;93(4):e2022284. https://doi.org/10.23750/abm.v93i4.12938	EXCLUDED—Article did not answer any research questions
35998965	David N	Mixed-methods investigation of barriers and needs in mental healthcare of adults with autism and recommendations for future care (BarrierfreeASD): study protocol	*BMJ Open.* 2022 Aug 23;12(8):e061773. https://doi.org/10.1136/bmjopen-2022-061773	EXCLUDED—This study was a protocol

(continued)

(continued)

PubMed ID	First author	Article title	Citation information	Reason why the citation was either included or excluded
35970662	Bevan S	Positive Healthcare Encounters for Children With Autism Spectrum Disorder: Accommodations During Surgical Procedures	*J Perianesth Nurs.* 2022 Aug 12:S1089-9472(22)00226-X. https://doi.org/10.1016/j.jopan.2022.05.070. Online ahead of print	EXCLUDED—Article did not answer any research questions
35969335	Gilmore D	Five Ways Providers Can Improve Mental Healthcare for Autistic Adults: A Review of Mental Healthcare Use, Barriers to Care, and Evidence-Based Recommendations	*Curr Psychiatry Rep.* 2022 Oct;24(10):565–571. https://doi.org/10.1007/s11920-022-01362-z. Epub 2022 Aug 15	EXCLUDED—Article did not answer any research questions
35854759	Stockham NT	An Informatics Analysis to Identify Sex Disparities and Healthcare Needs for Autism across the United States	*AMIA Annu Symp Proc.* 2022 May 23;2022:456–465. eCollection 2022	EXCLUDED—Article did not answer any research questions
35743364	Gabellone A	Expectations and Concerns about the Use of Telemedicine for Autism Spectrum Disorder: A Cross-Sectional Survey of Parents and Healthcare Professionals	*J Clin Med.* 2022 Jun 8;11(12):3294. https://doi.org/10.3390/jcm11123294	EXCLUDED—Article did not answer any research questions
35619147	Weir E	Autistic adults have poorer quality healthcare and worse health based on self-report data	*Mol Autism.* 2022 May 26;13(1):23. https://doi.org/10.1186/s13229-022-00501-w	INCLUDED—The study assessed prevalence of chronic health conditions, healthcare quality, differences in overall health inequality score, and effects of the coronavirus pandemic on healthcare quality

(continued)

(continued)

PubMed ID	First author	Article title	Citation information	Reason why the citation was either included or excluded
35561591	Joudar SS	Triage and priority-based healthcare diagnosis using artificial intelligence for autism spectrum disorder and gene contribution: A systematic review	*Comput Biol Med*. 2022 Jul;146:105553. https://doi.org/10.1016/j.compbiomed.2022.105553. Epub 2022 May 9	EXCLUDED—Article did not answer any research questions
35550238	Kang LRJ	A trial of the AASPIRE healthcare toolkit with Australian adults on the autism spectrum	*Aust J Prim Health*. 2022 Aug;28(4):350–356. https://doi.org/10.1071/PY21134	EXCLUDED—Article did not answer any research questions
35524328	Matin BK	Contributing factors to healthcare costs in individuals with autism spectrum disorder: a systematic review	*BMC Health Serv Res*. 2022 May 6;22(1):604. https://doi.org/10.1186/s12913-022-07932-4	EXCLUDED—Article did not answer any research questions
35498508	Angell AM	Effects of Sex, Race, and Ethnicity on Primary and Subspecialty Healthcare Use by Autistic Children in Florida: A Longitudinal Retrospective Cohort Study (2012–2018)	*Res Autism Spectr Disord*. 2022 Jun;94:101951. https://doi.org/10.1016/j.rasd.2022.101951. Epub 2022 Mar 21	EXCLUDED—Article did not answer any research questions
35313865	Moroe N	Rehabilitation healthcare professionals' competence and confidence in differentially diagnosing deafblindness from autism spectrum disorders: a cross-sectional survey in South Africa	*BMC Med Educ*. 2022 Mar 21;22(1):194. https://doi.org/10.1186/s12909-022-03258-1	EXCLUDED—Article did not answer any research questions

(continued)

(continued)

PubMed ID	First author	Article title	Citation information	Reason why the citation was either included or excluded
35285287	Cooper K	Healthcare clinician perspectives on the intersection of autism and gender dysphoria	*Autism.* 2022 Mar 14:13623613221080315. https://doi.org/10.1177/13623613221080315. Online ahead of print	EXCLUDED—Article did not answer any research questions
35262827	Ames JL	Opportunities for Inclusion and Engagement in the Transition of Autistic Youth from Pediatric to Adult Healthcare: A Qualitative Study	*J Autism Dev Disord.* 2022 Mar 9. https://doi.org/10.1007/s10803-022-05476-4. Online ahead of print	EXCLUDED—Article did not answer any research questions
35193921	Doherty M	Barriers to healthcare and self-reported adverse outcomes for autistic adults: a cross-sectional study	*BMJ Open.* 2022 Feb 22;12(2):e056904. https://doi.org/10.1136/bmjopen-2021-056904	INCLUDED—Our aim was to identify self-reported barriers to primary care access by autistic adults compared with non-autistic adults and to link these barriers to self-reported adverse health consequences
35165029	Myers RK	Transition to Adulthood for Autistic Adolescents: Topics Discussed by Healthcare Providers With Autistic Patients and Families	*J Adolesc Health.* 2022 May;70(5):829–832. https://doi.org/10.1016/j.jadohealth.2021.12.011. Epub 2022 Feb 11	EXCLUDED—Article did not answer any research questions
35126213	Aoki A	Trajectories of Healthcare Utilization Among Children and Adolescents With Autism Spectrum Disorder and/or Attention-Deficit/Hyperactivity Disorder in Japan	*Front Psychiatry.* 2022 Jan 20;12:812347. https://doi.org/10.3389/fpsyt.2021.812347. eCollection 2021	EXCLUDED—Article did not answer any research questions

(continued)

(continued)

PubMed ID	First author	Article title	Citation information	Reason why the citation was either included or excluded
35049626	Alenezi S	Burnout, Depression, and Anxiety Levels among Healthcare Workers Serving Children with Autism Spectrum Disorder	*Behav Sci (Basel)*. 2022 Jan 15;12(1):15. https://doi.org/10.3390/bs12010015	EXCLUDED—Article did not answer any research questions
34990000	Alain G	Expenditures and Healthcare Utilization of Patients Receiving Care at a Specialized Primary Care Clinic Designed with and for Autistic Adults	*J Gen Intern Med*. 2022 Aug;37(10):2413–2419. https://doi.org/10.1007/s11606-021-07180-y. Epub 2022 Jan 6	EXCLUDED—Article did not answer any research questions
34983217	Doherty M	Recognising autism in healthcare	*Br J Hosp Med (Lond)*. 2021 Dec 2;82(12):1–7. https://doi.org/10.12968/hmed.2021.0313. Epub 2021 Dec 8	EXCLUDED—Article did not answer any research questions
34983215	Haydon C	Autism: making reasonable adjustments in healthcare	*Br J Hosp Med (Lond)*. 2021 Dec 2;82(12):1–11. https://doi.org/10.12968/hmed.2021.0314. Epub 2021 Dec 8	EXCLUDED—Article did not answer any research questions
34906008	Calleja S	Barriers to Accessing Healthcare: Perspectives from Autistic Adults and Carers	*Qual Health Res*. 2022 Jan;32(2):267–278. https://doi.org/10.1177/10497323211050362. Epub 2021 Dec 14	INCLUDED—We conducted a qualitative analysis in Victoria (Australia) of the perceived experiences of healthcare access for autistic adults ($n = 9$) and primary caregivers of autistic adults ($n = 7$)
34881676	Gilmore D	Healthcare service use patterns among autistic adults: A systematic review with narrative synthesis	*Autism*. 2022 Feb;26(2):317–331. https://doi.org/10.1177/13623613211060906. Epub 2021 Dec 9	EXCLUDED—Article did not answer any research questions

(continued)

(continued)

PubMed ID	First author	Article title	Citation information	Reason why the citation was either included or excluded
34853958	Sartin EB	Brief Report: Healthcare Providers' Discussions Regarding Transportation and Driving with Autistic and Non-autistic Patients	*J Autism Dev Disord*. 2021 Dec 1:10.1007/s10803-021-05372-3. https://doi.org/10.1007/s10803-021-05372-3. Online ahead of print	EXCLUDED—Article did not answer any research questions
34825580	Lipinski S	A blind spot in mental healthcare? Psychotherapists lack education and expertise for the support of adults on the autism spectrum	*Autism*. 2022 Aug;26(6):1509–1521. https://doi.org/10.1177/13623613211057973. Epub 2021 Nov 26	EXCLUDED—Article did not answer any research questions
34320870	Snow SL	A balancing act: An interpretive description of healthcare providers' and families' perspective on the surgical experiences of children with autism spectrum disorder	*Autism*. 2022 May;26(4):839–848. https://doi.org/10.1177/13623613211034057. Epub 2021 Jul 28	EXCLUDED—Article did not answer any research questions
34232798	Wright Stein S	Understanding disability in healthcare: exploring the perceptions of parents of young people with autism spectrum disorder	*Disabil Rehabil*. 2022 Sep;44(19):5623–5630. https://doi.org/10.1080/09638288.2021.194 8114. Epub 2021 Jul 7	EXCLUDED—Article did not answer any research questions

(continued)

(continued)

PubMed ID	First author	Article title	Citation information	Reason why the citation was either included or excluded
34155717	Boshoff K	A meta-synthesis of how parents of children with autism describe their experience of accessing and using routine healthcare services for their children	*Health Soc Care Community*. 2021 Nov;29(6):1668–1682. https://doi.org/10.1111/hsc.13369. Epub 2021 Jun 21	INCLUDED—To bring greater understanding to parental experiences of supporting their child to access healthcare services, a systematic review of qualitative research was undertaken to address the following review question: 'How do parents of children with autism describe their experiences of utilising routine healthcare services?'
34037425	Hand BN	Healthcare utilization among children with early autism diagnoses, children with other developmental delays and a comparison group	*J Comp Eff Res*. 2021 Aug;10(11):917–926. https://doi.org/10.2217/cer-2021-0056. Epub 2021 May 26	EXCLUDED—Article did not answer any research questions
33977886	Sheehan R	Effects of the COVID-19 pandemic on mental healthcare and services: results of a UK survey of front-line staff working with people with intellectual disability and/or autism	*BJPsych Bull*. 2021 May 12:1–7. https://doi.org/10.1192/bjb.2021.52. Online ahead of print	EXCLUDED—Article did not answer any research questions

(continued)

(continued)

PubMed ID	First author	Article title	Citation information	Reason why the citation was either included or excluded
33910390	Mason D	How to improve healthcare for autistic people: A qualitative study of the views of autistic people and clinicians	*Autism.* 2021 Apr;25(3):774–785. https://doi. org/10.1177/1362361321993709	INCLUDED—This study investigated autistic people's experiences of healthcare and professionals' experiences of providing healthcare to autistic people
33876563	Srinivasan S	Needs assessment in unmet healthcare and family support services: A survey of caregivers of children and youth with autism spectrum disorder in Delaware	*Autism Res.* 2021 Aug;14(8):1736–1758. https://doi.org/10.1002/aur.2514. Epub 2021 Apr 19	EXCLUDED—Article did not answer any research questions
33767375	Malik-Soni N	Tackling healthcare access barriers for individuals with autism from diagnosis to adulthood	*Pediatr Res.* 2022 Apr;91(5):1028–1035. https://doi.org/10.1038/s41390-021-01465-y. Epub 2021 Mar 25	EXCLUDED—Article did not answer any research questions
33737429	Brice S	The importance and availability of adjustments to improve access for autistic adults who need mental and physical healthcare: findings from UK surveys	*BMJ Open.* 2021 Mar 18;11(3):e043336. https://doi.org/10.1136/bmjopen-2020-043336	INCLUDED—To investigate autistic people's views on the importance and availability of adjustments to mental and physical healthcare provision. To explore whether specific categories of adjustments can be identified and to identify any differences in their importance and availability between mental and physical healthcare

(continued)

(continued)

PubMed ID	First author	Article title	Citation information	Reason why the citation was either included or excluded
33588579	Babb C	'It's not that they don't want to access the support... it's the impact of the autism': The experience of eating disorder services from the perspective of autistic women, parents and healthcare professionals	*Autism*. 2021 Jul;25(5):1409–1421. https://doi.org/10.1177/1362361321991257. Epub 2021 Feb 15	EXCLUDED—Article did not answer any research questions
33402809	Sharma N	Comments on "Knowledge and Beliefs About Autism Spectrum Disorders in Indian Healthcare Professionals"	*Indian J Psychol Med*. 2020 Jul 13;42(4):405. https://doi.org/10.1177/0253717620930311. eCollection 2020 Jul	EXCLUDED—Article did not answer any research questions
33399017	McPherson AC	"It's not a simple answer." A qualitative study to explore how healthcare providers can best support families with a child with autism spectrum disorder and overweight or obesity	*Disabil Rehabil*. 2022 Jul;44(14):3540–3546. https://doi.org/10.1080/09638288.2020.1867909. Epub 2021 Jan 5	EXCLUDED—Article did not answer any research questions
33113106	Zuvekas SH	Healthcare Costs of Pediatric Autism Spectrum Disorder in the United States, 2003–2015	*J Autism Dev Disord*. 2021 Aug;51(8):2950–2958. https://doi.org/10.1007/s10803-020-04704-z.	EXCLUDED—Article did not answer any research questions
33103457	Nicolaidis C	Psychometric testing of a set of patient-reported instruments to assess healthcare interventions for autistic adults	*Autism*. 2021 Apr;25(3):786–799. https://doi.org/10.1177/1362361320967178. Epub 2020 Oct 25	EXCLUDED—Article did not answer any research questions

(continued)

(continued)

PubMed ID	First author	Article title	Citation information	Reason why the citation was either included or excluded
33072182	Walsh C	Development and evaluation of a novel caregiver-report tool to assess barriers to physical healthcare for people on the autism spectrum	*Res Autism Spectr Disord.* 2020 Nov;79:101,680. https://doi.org/10.1016/j.rasd.2020.101680. Epub 2020 Oct 14	EXCLUDED—Article did not answer any research questions
33044397	Cheak-Zamora N	Provider Perspectives on the Extension for Community Healthcare Outcomes Autism: Transition to Adulthood Program	*J Dev Behav Pediatr.* 2021 Feb–Mar 01;42(2):91–100. https://doi.org/10.1097/DBP.0000000000000872	EXCLUDED—Article did not answer any research questions
33004421	Clifford A	Patient and Family-Centred Care (PFCC) as an evidence-based framework for optimising the acute healthcare experiences of families of young people with autism	*Evid Based Nurs.* 2021 Oct;24(4):133. https://doi.org/10.1136/ebnurs-2020-103309. Epub 2020 Oct 1	EXCLUDED—Article did not answer any research questions
36112897	Walsh C	Barriers to Healthcare for Persons with Autism: A Systematic Review of the Literature and Development of a Taxonomy	*Dev Neurorehabil.* 2020 Oct;23(7):413–430. https://doi.org/10.1080/17518423.2020.171 6868. Epub 2020 Feb 6	EXCLUDED—This was a literature review that aimed to 1) synthesise extant research on barriers to healthcare access experienced by persons with autism, their caregivers, and healthcare providers; and 2) present a taxonomy of barriers to physical healthcare for individuals with autism
32859135	Nicolaidis C	Development and psychometric testing of the AASPIRE Adult Autism Healthcare Provider Self-Efficacy Scale	*Autism.* 2021 Apr;25(3):767–773. https://doi.org/10.1177/1362361320949734. Epub 2020 Aug 28	EXCLUDED—Article did not answer any research questions

(continued)

(continued)

PubMed ID	First author	Article title	Citation information	Reason why the citation was either included or excluded
32735419	Bellesheim KR	ECHO Autism: Integrating Maintenance of Certification with Extension for Community Healthcare Outcomes Improves Developmental Screening	*J Dev Behav Pediatr*. 2020 Aug;41(6):420–427. https://doi.org/10.1097/DBP.0000000000000796	EXCLUDED—Article did not answer any research questions
32702830	Calleja S	Healthcare access for autistic adults: A systematic review	*Medicine (Baltimore)*. 2020 Jul 17;99(29);e20899. https://doi.org/10.1097/MD.0000000000020899	EXCLUDED—This paper was a literature review
32583679	Ames JL	Healthcare service utilization and cost among transition-age youth with autism spectrum disorder and other special healthcare needs	*Autism*. 2021 Apr;25(3):705–718. https://doi.org/10.1177/1362361320931268. Epub 2020 Jun 25	EXCLUDED—Article did not answer any research questions
32332232	Kilmer M	Primary care of children with autism spectrum disorders: Developing confident healthcare leaders	*Nurse Pract*. 2020 May;45(5):41–47. https://doi.org/10.1097/01.NPR.0000660352.527 66.72	EXCLUDED—Article did not answer any research questions
32258436		Correction: investigating the association between early years foundation stage profile scores and subsequent diagnosis of an autism spectrum disorder: a retrospective study of linked healthcare and education data	*BMJ Paediatr Open*. 2020 Mar 23;4(1):e000483corr1. https://doi.org/10.1136/bmjpo-2019-000483corr1. eCollection 2020	EXCLUDED—This is a correction of a previous article
32202435	Norris JE	Interviewing autistic adults: Adaptations to support recall in police, employment, and healthcare interviews	*Autism*. 2020 Aug;24(6):1506–1520. https://doi.org/10.1177/1362361320909174. Epub 2020 Mar 23	EXCLUDED—Article did not answer any research questions

(continued)

(continued)

PubMed ID	First author	Article title	Citation information	Reason why the citation was either included or excluded
31799449	Wright B	Investigating the association between early years foundation stage profile scores and subsequent diagnosis of an autism spectrum disorder: a retrospective study of linked healthcare and education data	*BMJ Paediatr Open.* 2019 Nov 11;3(1):e000483. https://doi.org/10.1136/bmjpo-2019-000483. eCollection 2019	EXCLUDED—Article did not answer any research questions
31749388	Satkoske V	Autism and Advance Directives: Determining Capability and the Use of Health-Care Tools to Aid in Effective Communication and Decision-Making	*Am J Hosp Palliat Care.* 2020 May;37(5):354–363. https://doi.org/10.1177/1049909119888621. Epub 2019 Nov 21	EXCLUDED—Article did not answer any research questions
31727653	Tunesi S	Do autistic patients change healthcare services utilisation through the transition age? An Italian longitudinal retrospective study	*BMJ Open.* 2019 Nov 14;9(11):e030844. https://doi.org/10.1136/bmjopen-2019-030844	EXCLUDED—Article did not answer any research questions
31581793	Mazurek MO	ECHO Autism Transition: Enhancing healthcare for adolescents and young adults with autism spectrum disorder	*Autism.* 2020 Apr;24(3):633–644. https://doi.org/10.1177/1362361319879616. Epub 2019 Oct 3	EXCLUDED—Article did not answer any research questions
31440305	Wang L	Changes in Healthcare Expenditures After the Autism Insurance Mandate	*Res Autism Spectr Disord.* 2019 Jan;57:97–104. https://doi.org/10.1016/j.rasd.2018.10.004. Epub 2018 Oct 29	EXCLUDED—Article did not answer any research questions
31385792	Swetlik C	Adults with autism spectrum disorder: Updated considerations for healthcare providers	*Cleve Clin J Med.* 2019 Aug;86(8):543–553. https://doi.org/10.3949/ccjm.86a.18100	EXCLUDED—Article did not answer any research questions

(continued)

(continued)

PubMed ID	First author	Article title	Citation information	Reason why the citation was either included or excluded
31372123	Hayat AA	Assessment of knowledge about childhood autism spectrum disorder among healthcare workers in Makkah- Saudi Arabia	*Pak J Med Sci.* 2019 July–Aug;35(4):951–957. https://doi.org/10. 12669/pjms.35.4.605	EXCLUDED—Article did not answer any research questions
31352637	Jariwala-Parikh K	Autism Prevalence in the Medicaid Program and Healthcare Utilization and Costs Among Adult Enrollees Diagnosed with Autism	*Adm Policy Ment Health.* 2019 Nov;46(6):768–776. https://doi.org/10.1007/ s10488-019-00960-z	EXCLUDED—Article did not answer any research questions
31150751	McBain RK	Systematic Review: United States Workforce for Autism-Related Child Healthcare Services	*J Am Acad Child Adolesc Psychiatry.* 2020 Jan;59(1):113–139. https://doi.org/10.1016/j. jaac.2019.04.027. Epub 2019 May 29	EXCLUDED—Article did not answer any research questions
31124030	Mason D	A Systematic Review of What Barriers and Facilitators Prevent and Enable Physical Healthcare Services Access for Autistic Adults	*J Autism Dev Disord.* 2019 Aug;49(8):3387–3400. https://doi.org/10. 1007/s10803-019-04049-2	INCLUDED—This systematic review sought to identify studies that report on barriers and facilitators to physical healthcare access for autistic people
31044151	Giachetto G	Extension for Community Healthcare Outcomes Uruguay: A New Strategy to Promote Best Primary Care Practice for Autism	*Glob Pediatr Health.* 2019 Apr 2:6:2333794X19833734. https://doi.org/10. 1177/2333794X19833734. eCollection 2019	EXCLUDED—Article did not answer any research questions
30976456	Stadnick NA	A mixed methods study to adapt and implement integrated mental healthcare for children with autism spectrum disorder	*Pilot Feasibility Stud.* 2019 Mar 28;:5:51. https://doi.org/10.1186/s40814-019-0434-5. eCollection 2019	EXCLUDED—Article did not answer any research questions

(continued)

(continued)

PubMed ID	First author	Article title	Citation information	Reason why the citation was either included or excluded
30943759	Croteau C	Use, costs, and predictors of psychiatric healthcare services following an autism spectrum diagnosis: Population-based cohort study	*Autism*. 2019 Nov;23(8):2020–2030. https://doi.org/10.1177/1362361319840229. Epub 2019 Apr 4	EXCLUDED—Article did not answer any research questions
30762771	Calleja S	The disparities of healthcare access for adults with autism spectrum disorder: Protocol for a systematic review	*Medicine (Baltimore)*. 2019 Feb;98(7):e14480. https://doi.org/10.1097/MD.0000000000014480	EXCLUDED—This is a research protocol
30758692	Morris R	Healthcare Providers' Experiences with Autism: A Scoping Review	*J Autism Dev Disord*. 2019 Jun;49(6):2374–2388. https://doi.org/10.1007/s10803-019-03912-6	INCLUDED—A scoping review was conducted focusing on the experiences of healthcare professionals working with individuals with autism
30536218	Iannuzzi D	Addressing a Gap in Healthcare Access for Transition-Age Youth with Autism: A Pilot Educational Intervention for Family Nurse Practitioner Students	*J Autism Dev Disord*. 2019 Apr;49(4):1493–1504. https://doi.org/10.1007/s10803-018-3846-9	EXCLUDED—Article did not answer any research questions
30497274	Lindly OJ	Healthcare access and services use among US children with autism spectrum disorder	*Autism*. 2019 Aug;23(6):1419–1430. https://doi.org/10.1177/1362361318815237. Epub 2018 Nov 29	EXCLUDED—Article did not answer any research questions
30334893	Deon Kidd V	Preparing for Autistic Patients in Orthopaedic Surgery: Tips for a Successful Health-Care Interaction	*J Bone Joint Surg Am*. 2018 Oct 17;100(20):e132. https://doi.org/10.2106/JBJS.18.00252	EXCLUDED—Article did not answer any research questions

(continued)

(continued)

PubMed ID	First author	Article title	Citation information	Reason why the citation was either included or excluded
30220443	Berg KL	Adverse Childhood Experiences Are Associated with Unmet Healthcare Needs among Children with Autism Spectrum Disorder	*J Pediatr*. 2018 Nov;202:258–264.e1. https://doi.org/10.1016/j.jpeds.2018.07.021. Epub 2018 Sep 14	EXCLUDED—Article did not answer any research questions
30025674	Ofei SY	Constipation Burden in Children with Autism Spectrum Disorder: Emergency Department and Healthcare Use	*J Pediatr*. 2018 Nov;202:12–13. https://doi.org/10.1016/j.jpeds.2018.06.057. Epub 2018 Jul 17	EXCLUDED—Article did not answer any research questions
29485751	Gettis MA	Identifying Best Practice for Healthcare Providers Caring for Autistic Children Perioperatively	*Worldviews Evid Based Nurs*. 2018 Apr;15(2):127–129. https://doi.org/10.1111/wvn.12278. Epub 2018 Feb 27	EXCLUDED—Article did not answer any research questions

Note † This was a duplicate record

Appendix 2.1: Results of Studies Examined by Mason and Colleagues (2019)

Study	Population	Focus	Research type and study design	Findings
Nicolaidis et al. (2015)	39 autistic adults (who report an autism spectrum diagnosis); mean age 35 years (19–64) 16 supporters of an autistic person(s); mean age 52 years (28–74)	To obtain an in-depth understanding of autistic adults' experiences with healthcare and their recommendations for improving care	*Qualitative.* Individual interviews (participants could respond to questions via telephone, e-mail, or instant messenger); thematic analysis with an inductive approach at a semantic level	Identifies three clusters of barriers: patient-level factors (e.g., verbal communication skills, slow processing speed); provider-level factors (e.g., knowledge about autism in adults, use of accessible language); and system-level factors (e.g., availability of formal/informal support, stigma about autism)

(continued)

(continued)

Study	Population	Focus	Research type and study design	Findings
Dern and Sappok (2016)	Autistic self-advocates and autism professionals (sample size and composition are not described)	The available experiences of autism self-advocates and clinical experiences of practitioners	*Qualitative.* Summation of key meetings from a 5 year (2006–2011) series of meetings between autism self-advocates and healthcare professionals	Identifies barriers to healthcare for autistic people (i.e., difficulties making phone calls, lack of time to think/respond or use written notes). Recommends how professionals can improves healthcare for autistic adults (i.e., alternative methods to make appointments, allow patient to make notes/record discussions)

(continued)

(continued)

Study	Population	Focus	Research type and study design	Findings
Nicolaidis et al. (2016)	259 autistic adults who took part in cognitive interviews (n = 30, mean age 37.6 years, 20–64), test–retest reliability (n = 59, mean age 34.6, 18–64), pre- and post-intervention surveys (n = 170, mean age 36.5, 18–68); 51 primary care providers who took part in cognitive interviews (n = 10, mean age 41.6, 27–61), and a post-intervention survey (n = 41, mean age 36.3, 28–62)	Using community-based participatory research to create and evaluate an online healthcare toolkit for autistic adults and their primary care providers	*Mixed methodology.* Cognitive interviewing and test–retest studies. Toolkit evaluation was a single arm pre-/post-test intervention comparison of surveys with closed- and open-ended items	Almost all autistic participants and supporters rated the Toolkit as easy to use, important, and useful Most primary care providers rated the Toolkit as moderately or very useful and indicated they would recommend it to their patients Over the course of the intervention the number of self-reported barriers to healthcare reduced significantly from a mean of 4.1 to 2.8 (with healthcare self-efficacy scores also increasing significantly from 37.9 to 39.4 and satisfaction with patient-provider communication scores increasing significantly from 30.9 to 32.6)

(continued)

(continued)

Study	Population	Focus	Research type and study design	Findings
Raymaker et al. (2017)	209 autistic adults (mean age 37 years, SD = 13); 55 adults in a disability group (mean age 45, SD = 14); 174 adults in a non-autistic non-disabled group (mean age 38, SD = 12)	Identify and compare barriers to accessing healthcare experienced by autistic adults and adults with, and without other disabilities	*Quantitative*. Cross-sectional instrument development and validation (Long- and Short-Form Barriers to Healthcare Checklist)	Autistic adults and adults with other disabilities endorsed significantly more barriers than the non-autistic adults without disabilities. Autistic adults selected a different pattern and a greater number of barriers that adults with other disabilities, particularly in areas related to emotional regulation, patient-provider communication, sensory sensitivity, and healthcare navigation

(continued)

(continued)

Study	Population	Focus	Research type and study design	Findings
Vogan et al. (2017)	40 autistic adults (mean age 35.9, SD = 11.7)	Autistic adults access of healthcare services, experiences of accessing healthcare services, barriers to service use, and reported unmet service needs	*Quantitative.* Longitudinal study over a 12–18-month time frame, with participants completing measures every two months	The most commonly reported barriers by participants were not knowing where to find help (65.8%), overwhelming steps to seek help (52.6%), and negative experiences with professionals (47.4%). Over 75% endorsed three or more barriers to healthcare. Those with medical problems reported significantly more barriers to healthcare than those without (5.12, SD = 2.65; 3.20, SD = 2.25 respectively)

(continued)

(continued)

Study	Population	Focus	Research type and study design	Findings
Saqr et al. (2018)	126 autistic adults who took part in a retrospective chart analysis (mean age 21.2, SD = 5.6); 10 autistic adults who took part in a focus group (ages 18–30)	Environmental and process barriers to care access in a primary care setting and to examine medication use in the sample	*Mixed methodology.* Cross-sectional retrospective chart analysis; focus group	74 individualised plans were created for patients. The most common adjustment was taking the patient to the examination room upon arrival and completing registration there ($n = 16$) Focus group data highlighted the most stressful parts of the healthcare visit: waiting (both in the waiting room and examination room, and the examination). Furthermore, a negative feedback loop (fear of social interaction, heightens anxiety and overstimulation which makes social interaction difficult) was identified

Source Mason, D., Ingham, B., Urbanowicz, A., Michael, C., Birtles, H., Woodbury-Smith, M., Brown, T., James, I., Scarlett, C., Nicolaidis, C., & Parr, J. R. (2019). A Systematic Review of What Barriers and Facilitators Prevent and Enable Physical Healthcare Services Access for Autistic Adults. *Journal of Autism and Developmental Disorders, 49*(8), 3387–3400. https://doi.org/10.1007/s10803-019-040 49-2

References

Dern, S., & Sappok, T. (2016). Barriers to healthcare for people on the autism spectrum. *Advances in Autism*, *2*(1), 2–11. https://doi.org/10.1108/AIA-10-2015-0020

Nicolaidis, C., Raymaker, D. M., Ashkenazy, E., McDonald, K. E., Dern, S., Baggs, A. E., Kapp, S. K., Weiner, M., & Boisclair, W. C. (2015). "Respect the way I need to communicate with you": Healthcare experiences of adults on the autism spectrum. *Autism: The International Journal of Research and Practice*, *19*(7), 824–831. https://doi.org/10.1177/1362361315576221

Nicolaidis, C., Raymaker, D., McDonald, K., Kapp, S., Weiner, M., Ashkenazy, E., Gerrity, M., Kripke, C., Platt, L., & Baggs, A. (2016). The Development and Evaluation of an Online Healthcare Toolkit for Autistic Adults and their Primary Care Providers. *Journal of General Internal Medicine*, *31*(10), 1180–1189. https://doi.org/10.1007/s11606-016-3763-6

Raymaker, D. M., McDonald, K. E., Ashkenazy, E., Gerrity, M., Baggs, A. M., Kripke, C., Hourston, S., & Nicolaidis, C. (2017). Barriers to healthcare: Instrument development and comparison between autistic adults and adults with and without other disabilities. *Autism: The International Journal of Research and Practice*, *21*(8), 972–984. https://doi.org/10.1177/1362361316661261

Saqr, Y., Braun, E., Porter, K., Barnette, D., & Hanks, C. (2018). Addressing medical needs of adolescents and adults with autism spectrum disorders in a primary care setting. *Autism: The International Journal of Research and Practice*, *22*(1), 51–61. https://doi.org/10.1177/136236 1317709970

Vogan, V., Lake, J. K., Tint, A., Weiss, J. A., & Lunsky, Y. (2017). Tracking health care service use and the experiences of adults with autism spectrum disorder without intellectual disability: A longitudinal study of service rates, barriers and satisfaction. *Disability and Health Journal*, *10*(2), 264–270. https://doi.org/10.1016/j.dhjo.2016.11.002

Appendix 2.2: Healthcare Satisfaction Survey

Differences in sensory processing

Do you have any differences in sensory processing as compared with others (e.g. to light/visual cues, sound, touch, smell, etc. …)?

- Yes ☐
- No ☐

If yes, please select all that apply:

- One or more of my sense are heightened, as compared with others ☐
- One or more of my senses are muted, as compared with others ☐

Please answer the following questions about your experiences of going to see a healthcare professional (Doctor, General Practitioner, Nurse Practitioner, Nurse, or Physician's Assistant)

	Definitely agree	Slightly agree	Slightly disagree	Definitely disagree
I was able to describe how my symptoms felt in my body	☐	☐	☐	☐

(continued)

(continued)

	Definitely agree	Slightly agree	Slightly disagree	Definitely disagree
I was able to describe how bad my pain felt	☐	☐	☐	☐
I was able to describe my sensory processing difficulties to healthcare professionals	☐	☐	☐	☐
The sensory environment of the **waiting room** was more overwhelming than other environments	☐	☐	☐	☐
The sensory environment of the **examination room** was more overwhelming than other environments	☐	☐	☐	☐
My senses frequently overwhelm me so that I had trouble focusing on conversations with healthcare professionals	☐	☐	☐	☐

Communication during the healthcare consultation

Please answer the following questions about your experiences of going to see a healthcare professional (Doctor, General Practitioner, Nurse Practitioner, Nurse, or Physician's Assistant)

	Definitely agree	Slightly agree	Slightly disagree	Definitely disagree
I was able to explain what my symptoms were	☐	☐	☐	☐
I understood what my healthcare provider meant when they discussed my health	☐	☐	☐	☐
I did not ask all the questions I would like to about my health	☐	☐	☐	☐
I could explain my health concerns even if my healthcare professional did not ask me about them	☐	☐	☐	☐
I knew what was expected of me when I went to see my healthcare professional	☐	☐	☐	☐

Anxiety from healthcare experiences

Please answer the following questions about your experiences of going to see a healthcare professional (Doctor, General Practitioner, Nurse Practitioner, Nurse, or Physician's Assistant)

	Definitely agree	Slightly agree	Slightly disagree	Definitely disagree
The idea of going to see a healthcare professional made me feel anxious	☐	☐	☐	☐
The environment of the **waiting room** and/or the **examination room** made me feel anxious	☐	☐	☐	☐
I feel anxious when I saw a different healthcare professional to whom I expect	☐	☐	☐	☐
The process of setting up an appointment made me feel anxious	☐	☐	☐	☐
I frequently leave my healthcare professional's office feeling as thought I did not receive any help at all	☐	☐	☐	☐

System problems regarding healthcare

Please answer the following questions about your experiences of going to see a healthcare professional (Doctor, General Practitioner, Nurse Practitioner, Nurse, or Physician's Assistant)

	Definitely agree	Slightly agree	Slightly disagree	Definitely disagree
In most appointments, I had enough time to discuss my concerns with healthcare professionals	☐	☐	☐	☐
If I need to go to see a specialist for a healthcare concern, I can do so	☐	☐	☐	☐
I often choose not to go to the doctor with concerns if I need to see a specialist because I know that it will take me many appointments before I can see the specialist	☐	☐	☐	☐
I usually leave my appointments knowing what the next steps are (i.e., follow-up appointments, medications, etc.)	☐	☐	☐	☐
I am provided with appropriate support after I receive a diagnosis of any kind (i.e., anything from infections to chronic conditions)	☐	☐	☐	☐

Source Weir, E., Allison, C., & Baron-Cohen, S. (2022). Autistic adults have poorer quality healthcare and worse health based on self-report data. *Molecular Autism*, *13*(1), 23. https://doi.org/10.1186/s13229-022-00501-w

Appendix 2.3: My Healthcare Needs

Personal information

My name is: _____

I would like you to call me: _____

My date of birth is (Day/Month/Year): _____/ _____/ _____
Emergency contact information

If an emergency happens, I would like the doctor/dentist to contact the following person

Name: _____

Their relationship to me: _____

Their phone number is: _____
Another person that the doctor/dentist can contact is

Name: _____

Their relationship to me: _____

Their phone number is: _____
My medications

Question	Yes	No
I take medications	☐	☐
If yes, I take the following medications:		

Please talk to this person before changing my medication

Name: _____

Their relationship to me: _____

Their phone number is: _____

How staff can communicate with me

Question	Yes	No
Can the doctor/dentist ask me questions?	☐	☐
I would like the doctor/dentist to ask me short and very specific questions	☐	☐
I would like the doctor/dentist to write things down for me	☐	☐
I would prefer symbols and/or pictures	☐	☐
I would like my doctor/dentist to demonstrate things	☐	☐
I would like my doctor/dentist to give me a lot of time to think about their questions	☐	☐
I would like my carer to explain what the doctor/dentist is asking me	☐	☐

How I will communicate with healthcare staff

Question	Yes	No
I will talk to the doctor/dentist	☐	☐
I would like to write my answers	☐	☐
I would like to use pictures or symbols to explain things	☐	☐
I would like to demonstrate things	☐	☐
I would like my carer to answer questions for me	☐	☐

How I explain pain and discomfort

Question	Yes	No
When I feel physical pain I:		
Scream	☐	☐
Run away	☐	☐
Fight	☐	☐
Other behaviours:		

How I communicate my physical pain to others

Question	Yes	No
I can tell the healthcare staff that I have physical pain	☐	☐
I will talk to the healthcare staff about my physical pain	☐	☐
I can point to the physical pain that my body feels	☐	☐
I become very quiet and withdrawn when I feel physical pain	☐	☐
I become very upset and maybe even angry or aggressive when I feel physical pain	☐	☐

<u>Things that cause me discomfort/distress</u>

Question	Yes	No
I do not like people getting too close to me	☐	☐
I become distressed or uncomfortable when people physically touch me	☐	☐
I find the smells or feel of rubber gloves unpleasant	☐	☐
Hard and cold medical/dental equipment will be uncomfortable for me	☐	☐
I do not like bright lights shining in my eyes	☐	☐
I do not like tight things touching my body (e.g., blood pressure cuffs)	☐	☐
I dislike giving blood samples	☐	☐
I feel uncomfortable being in a confined/enclosed space (e.g., being in a body scanner)	☐	☐
I have difficulty swallowing tablets	☐	☐

<u>Strategies that can help me avoid stress</u>

Question	Yes	No
If I am warned and supported, I can cope with bright lights	☐	☐
If I am warned and supported, I can cope with noises that make me feel uneasy	☐	☐
If I am warned and supported, I can cope with tight-fitting medical equipment (e.g., blood pressure cuffs)	☐	☐
I can give a blood sample if I am warned and supported (e.g., given anesthetic cream at the injection site)	☐	☐
If I am warned and supported, I can cope with enclosed spaces	☐	☐

<u>Other things that I would like you to know about me</u>

Issues I might have	Explanation
Sensory needs	
Special interests	
Things that make me feel happy	

Source National Autistic Society. (2023). *My Health Passport for autistic people.* https://dy55nn drxke1w.cloudfront.net/file/24/.ZuLn47.Z3Oq7eJ.ZkJp.0QsoHD/Health_Passport_A4_Editable_2022.pdf

Printed by Printforce, the Netherlands